This report contains the collective views of an international group of experts and does not necessarily represent the decisions or the stated policy of the United Nations Environment Programme, the International Labour Organisation, or the World Health Organization

Environmental Health Criteria 195

HEXACHLOROBENZENE

First draft prepared by Mr R. Newhook and Ms W. Dormer,
Health Canada, Canada

Published under the joint sponsorship of the United Nations Environment Programme, the International Labour Organisation, and the World Health Organization, and produced within the framework of the Inter-Organization Programme for the Sound Management of Chemicals.

World Health Organization
Geneva, 1997

The **International Programme on Chemical Safety (IPCS)**, established in 1980, is a joint venture of the United Nations Environment Programme (UNEP), the International Labour Organisation (ILO), and the World Health Organization (WHO). The overall objectives of the IPCS are to establish the scientific basis for assessment of the risk to human health and the environment from exposure to chemicals, through international peer-review processes, as a prerequisite for the promotion of chemical safety, and to provide technical assistance in strengthening national capacities for the sound management of chemicals.

The **Inter-Organization Programme for the Sound Management of Chemicals (IOMC)** was established in 1995 by UNEP, ILO, the Food and Agriculture Organization of the United Nations, WHO, the United Nations Industrial Development Organization and the Organisation for Economic Co-operation and Development (Participating Organizations), following recommendations made by the 1992 UN Conference on Environment and Development to strengthen cooperation and increase coordination in the field of chemical safety. The purpose of the IOMC is to promote coordination of the policies and activities pursued by the Participating Organizations, jointly or separately, to achieve the sound management of chemicals in relation to human health and the environment.

WHO Library Cataloguing in Publication Data

Hexachlorobenzene.

(Environmental health criteria ; 195)

1.Hexachlorobenzene - toxicity 2.Hexachlorobenzene - adverse effects
3.Environmental exposure I.Series

ISBN 92 4 157195 0 (NLM Classification: QV 633)
ISSN 0250-863X

PRINTED IN FINLAND
97/11662 – VAMMALA – 5000

CONTENTS

ENVIRONMENTAL HEALTH CRITERIA FOR HEXACHLOROBENZENE

NOTE TO READERS OF THE CRITERIA MONOGRAPHS

Every effort has been made to present information in the criteria monographs as accurately as possible without unduly delaying their publication. In the interest of all users of the Environmental Health Criteria monographs, readers are requested to communicate any errors that may have occurred to the Director of the International Programme on Chemical Safety, World Health Organization, Geneva, Switzerland, in order that they may be included in corrigenda.

* * *

A detailed data profile and a legal file can be obtained from the International Register of Potentially Toxic Chemicals, Case postale 356, 1219 Châtelaine, Geneva, Switzerland (telephone no. + 41 22 - 9799111, fax no. + 41 22 - 7973460, E-mail irptc@unep.ch).

* * *

This publication was made possible by grant number 5 U01 ES02617-15 from the National Institute of Environmental Health Sciences, National Institutes of Health, USA, and by financial support from the European Commission and the Federal Ministry for the Environment, Nature Conservation and Nuclear Safety, Germany.

Environmental Health Criteria

P R E A M B L E

Objectives

In 1973 the WHO Environmental Health Criteria Programme was initiated with the following objectives:

(i) to assess information on the relationship between exposure to environmental pollutants and human health, and to provide guidelines for setting exposure limits;

(ii) to identify new or potential pollutants;

(iii) to identify gaps in knowledge concerning the health effects of pollutants;

(iv) to promote the harmonization of toxicological and epidemiological methods in order to have internationally comparable results.

The first Environmental Health Criteria (EHC) monograph, on mercury, was published in 1976 and since that time an ever-increasing number of assessments of chemicals and of physical effects have been produced. In addition, many EHC monographs have been devoted to evaluating toxicological methodology, e.g., for genetic, neurotoxic, teratogenic and nephrotoxic effects. Other publications have been concerned with epidemiological guidelines, evaluation of short-term tests for carcinogens, biomarkers, effects on the elderly and so forth.

Since its inauguration the EHC Programme has widened its scope, and the importance of environmental effects, in addition to health effects, has been increasingly emphasized in the total evaluation of chemicals.

The original impetus for the Programme came from World Health Assembly resolutions and the recommendations of the 1972 UN Conference on the Human Environment. Subsequently the work became an integral part of the International Programme on Chemical Safety (IPCS), a cooperative programme of UNEP, ILO and WHO. In this manner, with the strong support of the new partners, the importance of occupational health and environmental effects was fully recognized. The EHC monographs have become widely established, used and recognized throughout the world.

The recommendations of the 1992 UN Conference on Environment and Development and the subsequent establishment of the Intergovernmental Forum on Chemical Safety with the priorities for action in the six programme areas of Chapter 19, Agenda 21, all lend further weight to the need for EHC assessments of the risks of chemicals.

Scope

The criteria monographs are intended to provide critical reviews on the effect on human health and the environment of chemicals and of combinations of chemicals and physical and biological agents. As such, they include and review studies that are of direct relevance for the evaluation. However, they do not describe *every* study carried out. Worldwide data are used and are quoted from original studies, not from abstracts or reviews. Both published and unpublished reports are considered and it is incumbent on the authors to assess all the articles cited in the references. Preference is always given to published data. Unpublished data are only used when relevant published data are absent or when they are pivotal to the risk assessment. A detailed policy statement is available that describes the procedures used for unpublished proprietary data so that this information can be used in the evaluation without compromising its confidential nature (WHO (1990) Revised Guidelines for the Preparation of Environmental Health Criteria Monographs. PCS/90.69, Geneva, World Health Organization).

In the evaluation of human health risks, sound human data, whenever available, are preferred to animal data. Animal and *in vitro* studies provide support and are used mainly to supply evidence missing from human studies. It is mandatory that research on human subjects is conducted in full accord with ethical principles, including the provisions of the Helsinki Declaration.

The EHC monographs are intended to assist national and international authorities in making risk assessments and subsequent risk management decisions. They represent a thorough evaluation of risks and are not, in any sense, recommendations for regulation or standard setting. These latter are the exclusive purview of national and regional governments.

Content

The layout of EHC monographs for chemicals is outlined below.

- Summary - a review of the salient facts and the risk evaluation of the chemical
- Identity - physical and chemical properties, analytical methods
- Sources of exposure
- Environmental transport, distribution and transformation
- Environmental levels and human exposure
- Kinetics and metabolism in laboratory animals and humans
- Effects on laboratory mammals and *in vitro* test systems
- Effects on humans
- Effects on other organisms in the laboratory and field
- Evaluation of human health risks and effects on the environment
- Conclusions and recommendations for protection of human health and the environment
- Further research
- Previous evaluations by international bodies, e.g., IARC, JECFA, JMPR

Selection of chemicals

Since the inception of the EHC Programme, the IPCS has organized meetings of scientists to establish lists of priority chemicals for subsequent evaluation. Such meetings have been held in: Ispra, Italy, 1980; Oxford, United Kingdom, 1984; Berlin, Germany, 1987; and North Carolina, USA, 1995. The selection of chemicals has been based on the following criteria: the existence of scientific evidence that the substance presents a hazard to human health and/or the environment; the possible use, persistence, accumulation or degradation of the substance shows that there may be significant human or environmental exposure; the size and nature of populations at risk (both human and other species) and risks for environment;

international concern, i.e. the substance is of major interest to several countries; adequate data on the hazards are available.

If an EHC monograph is proposed for a chemical not on the priority list, the IPCS Secretariat consults with the Cooperating Organizations and all the Participating Institutions before embarking on the preparation of the monograph.

Procedures

The order of procedures that result in the publication of an EHC monograph is shown in the flow chart. A designated staff member of IPCS, responsible for the scientific quality of the document, serves as Responsible Officer (RO). The IPCS Editor is responsible for layout and language. The first draft, prepared by consultants or, more usually, staff from an IPCS Participating Institution, is based initially on data provided from the International Register of Potentially Toxic Chemicals, and reference data bases such as Medline and Toxline.

The draft document, when received by the RO, may require an initial review by a small panel of experts to determine its scientific quality and objectivity. Once the RO finds the document acceptable as a first draft, it is distributed, in its unedited form, to well over 150 EHC contact points throughout the world who are asked to comment on its completeness and accuracy and, where necessary, provide additional material. The contact points, usually designated by governments, may be Participating Institutions, IPCS Focal Points, or individual scientists known for their particular expertise. Generally some four months are allowed before the comments are considered by the RO and author(s). A second draft incorporating comments received and approved by the Director, IPCS, is then distributed to Task Group members, who carry out the peer review, at least six weeks before their meeting.

The Task Group members serve as individual scientists, not as representatives of any organization, government or industry. Their function is to evaluate the accuracy, significance and relevance of the information in the document and to assess the health and environmental risks from exposure to the chemical. A summary and

EHC PREPARATION FLOW CHART

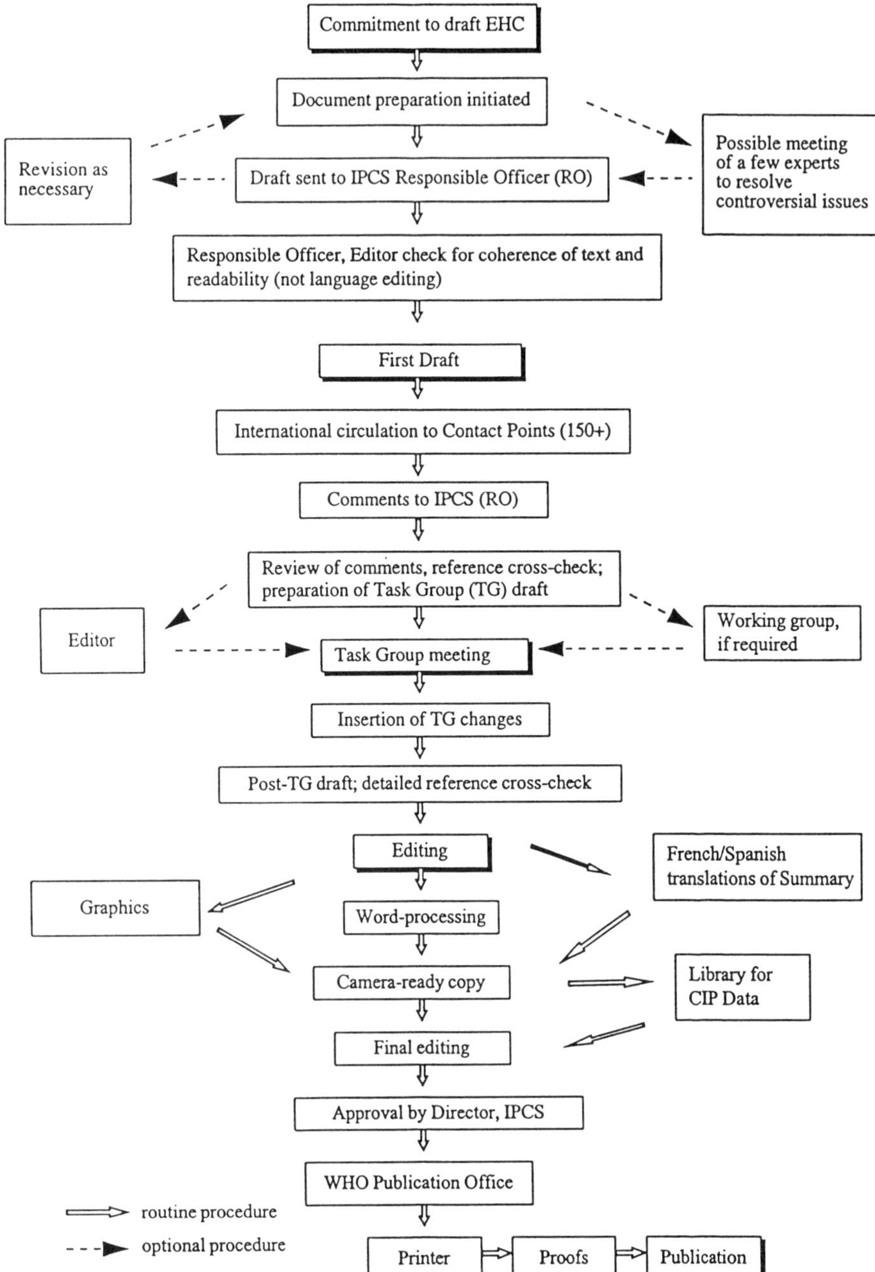

recommendations for further research and improved safety aspects are also required. The composition of the Task Group is dictated by the range of expertise required for the subject of the meeting and by the need for a balanced geographical distribution.

The three cooperating organizations of the IPCS recognize the important role played by nongovernmental organizations. Representatives from relevant national and international associations may be invited to join the Task Group as observers. While observers may provide a valuable contribution to the process, they can only speak at the invitation of the Chairperson. Observers do not participate in the final evaluation of the chemical; this is the sole responsibility of the Task Group members. When the Task Group considers it to be appropriate, it may meet *in camera*.

All individuals who as authors, consultants or advisers participate in the preparation of the EHC monograph must, in addition to serving in their personal capacity as scientists, inform the RO if at any time a conflict of interest, whether actual or potential, could be perceived in their work. They are required to sign a conflict of interest statement. Such a procedure ensures the transparency and probity of the process.

When the Task Group has completed its review and the RO is satisfied as to the scientific correctness and completeness of the document, it then goes for language editing, reference checking, and preparation of camera-ready copy. After approval by the Director, IPCS, the monograph is submitted to the WHO Office of Publications for printing. At this time a copy of the final draft is sent to the Chairperson and Rapporteur of the Task Group to check for any errors.

It is accepted that the following criteria should initiate the updating of an EHC monograph: new data are available that would substantially change the evaluation; there is public concern for health or environmental effects of the agent because of greater exposure; an appreciable time period has elapsed since the last evaluation.

All Participating Institutions are informed, through the EHC progress report, of the authors and institutions proposed for the drafting of the documents. A comprehensive file of all comments received on drafts of each EHC monograph is maintained and is available on request. The Chairpersons of Task Groups are briefed before each meeting on their role and responsibility in ensuring that these rules are followed.

WHO TASK GROUP ON ENVIRONMENTAL HEALTH CRITERIA FOR HEXACHLOROBENZENE

Members

Dr D. Arnold, Health Canada, Tunney's Pasture, Ottawa, Ontario Canada

Dr A. Göcmen, Department of Pediatrics, Faculty of Medicine, Hacettepe University, Hacettepe, Ankara, Turkey

Professor B. Jansson, Institute of Applied Environmental Research, ITM-Solna, Stockholm University, Stockholm, Sweden

Dr J. Jarrell, Foothills Hospital, Calgary Regional Health Authority, Calgary, Alberta, Canada

Dr A. Langley, South Australian Health Commission, Rundle Mall, Australia (*Chairman*)

Mr R. Newhook, Bureau of Chemical Hazards, Environmental Substances Division, Health Canada, Tunney's Pasture, Ottawa, Ontario, Canada (*Rapporteur*)

Dr D. Peakall, Wimbledon, London, United Kingdom (*Vice-chairman*)

Dr A.G. Smith, Medical Research Council Toxicology Unit, Hodgkin Building, University of Leicester, Leicester, United Kingdom

Dr J. Sunyer, Department of Epidemiology and Public Health, Institut Municipal d'Investigacio Medica, Barcelona, Spain

Dr A. van Birgelen, National Health and Environmental Effects Research Laboratory, Pharmacokinetics Branch, US Environmental Protection Agency, Research Triangle Park, North Carolina, USA[a]

Dr J. Vos, National Institute of Public Health and the Environment (RIVM), Hygiene, Bilthoven, The Netherlands

Observers

Dr J. de Gerlache, Solvay SA, Department of Chemical Safety and Toxicology, Brussels, Belgium (Representing EURO CHLOR)

Dr Roger Drew, Toxicology Information Section, Safety, Health & Environment Division, ICI Australia Operations Pty Ltd., ICI House, Melbourne, Victoria, Australia (Representing European Centre for Ecotoxicology and Toxicology of Chemicals)

Secretariat

Dr G.C. Becking, Interregional Research Unit, International Programme on Chemical Safety, Research Triangle Park, North Carolina USA (*Secretary*)

Ms W. Dormer, Bureau of Chemical Hazards, Environmental Substances Division, Health Canada, Tunney's Pasture, Ottawa, Ontario, Canada (*Temporary Adviser to Secretariat*)

Dr J. Wilbourn, Unit of Carcinogen Identification and Evaluation, International Agency for Research on Cancer, Lyon, France

---

[a] Dr A. Van Birgelen's present address: National Institute of Environmental Health Sciences, Research Triangle Park, North Carolina, USA

IPCS TASK GROUP ON ENVIRONMENTAL HEALTH CRITERIA FOR HEXACHLOROBENZENE

A WHO Task Group on Environmental Health Criteria for Hexachlorobenzene met in Geneva from 26 February to 1 March 1996. Dr G.C. Becking, IPCS, welcomed the participants on behalf of Dr M. Mercier, Director of the IPCS, and the three cooperating organizations (UNEP/ILO/WHO). The group reviewed and revised the draft and made an evaluation of the risks for human health and the environment from exposure to hexachlorobenzene.

The first draft was prepared by Mr R. Newhook and Ms W. Dormer, Health Canada, Ottawa, Canada. These authors also prepared the draft reviewed by the Task Group, which incorporated the comments received following circulation of the first draft to IPCS Contact Points for Environmental Health Criteria monographs.

The IPCS gratefully acknowledges the financial and other support of the Health Protection Branch, Health Canada. This support was indispensable for the completion of this monograph.

Dr G.C. Becking (IPCS, Central Unit, Inter-regional Research Unit) and Dr P.G. Jenkins (IPCS, Central Unit, Geneva) were responsible for the overall scientific content and the technical editing, respectively, of this monograph.

The efforts of all who helped in the preparation and finalization of this publication are gratefully acknowledged.

ABBREVIATIONS

BCF	bioconcentration factor
BMF	biomagnification factor
DL	detection limit
HCB	hexachlorobenzene
i.p.	intraperitoneal
ND	not detectable
PCT	porphyria cutanea tarda
p,p'DDE	1,1'-(2,2-dichloroethylidene)-bis[4-chlorobenzene]
SER	smooth endoplasmic reticulum
T_3	triiodothyronine
T_4	thyroxine

PREFACE

The preparation of comprehensive Environmental Health Criteria (EHC), as outlined in the Preamble of this monograph, is an extremely time-consuming and resource-intensive procedure. Often countries have prepared recent comprehensive reviews on chemicals as required by their national legislation, and the International Programme on Chemical Safety (IPCS) has been asked by Member States to determine how best to utilize such national reviews during the preparation of international EHC. Utilizing such national documents should avoid duplication of effort and result in the more rapid production of more concise IPCS EHC monographs.

This monograph on hexachlorobenzene has been prepared using as background document the review (Supporting Document) prepared under the Canadian Environmental Protection Act (CEPA), dated June 1993. From this document, staff of Health Canada have chosen only the most relevant studies for assessing the human and environmental risks from exposure to hexachlorobenzene. These have been described from the original references and supplemented by additional information published more recently. This has resulted in a concise monograph, yet one that supplies sufficient information for the reader to understand the basis for the conclusions reached by the Task Group.

Readers who wish to consult the text of the Canadian Supporting Document can obtain a copy from the Director, IPCS, World Health Organization, Geneva, Switzerland.

1. SUMMARY AND CONCLUSIONS

1.1 Identity, physical and chemical properties, and analytical methods

Hexachlorobenzene (HCB) is a chlorinated organic compound with moderate volatility. It is practically insoluble in water, but is highly lipid-soluble and bioaccumulative. Technical grade HCB contains up to 2% impurities, most of which is pentachlorobenzene. The remainder includes the higher chlorinated dibenzo-*p*-dioxins, dibenzofurans and biphenyls. Analysis of HCB in environmental media and biological materials generally involves extraction of the sample into organic solvents, often followed by a clean-up step, to produce organic extracts for gas chromatography/mass spectrometry (GC/MS) or gas chromatography with electron capture detection (GC/ECD).

1.2 Sources of human and environmental exposure

HCB was at one time used extensively as a seed dressing to prevent fungal disease on grains, but this use was discontinued in most countries in the 1970s. HCB continues to be released to the environment from a number of sources, including the use of some chlorinated pesticides, incomplete combustion, old dump sites and inappropriate manufacture and disposal of wastes from the manufacture of chlorinated solvents, chlorinated aromatics and chlorinated pesticides.

1.3 Environmental transport, distribution and transformation

HCB is distributed throughout the environment because it is mobile and persistent, although slow photodegradation in air and microbial degradation in soil do occur. In the troposphere, HCB is transported long distances and removed from the air phase through deposition to soil and water. Significant biomagnification of HCB through the food chain has been reported.

1.4 Environmental levels and human exposure

Low concentrations of HCB are present in ambient air (a few ng/m^3 or less) and in drinking-water and surface water (a few ng/litre or less) in areas that are distant from point sources around the world. However, higher levels have been measured near point sources. HCB is bioaccumulative and has been detected in invertebrates, fish, reptiles, birds and mammals (including humans) distant from point sources, particularly in fatty tissues of organisms at higher trophic levels. Mean levels in adipose tissue of the human general population in various countries range from tens to hundreds of ng/g wet weight. Based on representative levels of HCB in air, water and food, the total intake of HCB by adults in the general population is estimated to be between 0.0004 and 0.003 µg/kg body weight per day. This intake is predominantly from the diet. Owing to the presence of HCB in breast milk, mean intakes by nursing infants have been estimated to range from < 0.018 to 5.1 µg/kg body weight per day in various countries. The results of most studies on the levels of HCB in foods and human tissues over time indicate that exposure of the general population to HCB declined from the 1970s to the mid-1990s in many locations. However, this trend has not been evident during the last decade in some other locations.

1.5 Kinetics and metabolism in laboratory animals and humans

There is a lack of toxicokinetic information for humans. HCB is readily absorbed by the oral route in experimental animals and poorly via the skin (there are no data concerning inhalation). In animals and humans, HCB accumulates in lipid-rich tissues, such as adipose tissue, adrenal cortex, bone marrow, skin and some endocrine tissues, and can be transferred to offspring both across the placenta and via mothers' milk. HCB undergoes limited metabolism, yielding pentachlorophenol, tetrachlorohydroquinone and pentachlorothiophenol as the major metabolites in urine. Elimination half-lives for HCB range from approximately one month in rats and rabbits to 2 or 3 years in monkeys.

1.6 Effects on laboratory animals and *in vitro* tests

The acute toxicity of HCB to experimental animals is low (1000 to 10 000 mg/kg body weight). In animal studies, HCB is not a skin or eye irritant and does not sensitize the guinea-pig.

The available data on the systemic toxicity of HCB indicate that the pathway for the biosynthesis of haem is a major target of hexachlorobenzene toxicity. Elevated levels of porphyrins and/or porphyrin precursors have been found in the liver, other tissues and excreta of several species of laboratory mammals exposed to HCB. Porphyria has been reported in a number of studies in rats with subchronic or chronic oral exposure to between 2.5 and 15 mg HCB/kg body weight per day. Excretion of coproporphyrins was increased in pigs ingesting 0.5 mg HCB/kg body weight per day or more (no effects were observed at 0.05 mg HCB/kg body weight per day in the latter study). Repeated exposure to HCB has also been shown to affect a wide range of organ systems (including the liver, lungs, kidneys, thyroid, skin, and nervous and immune systems), although these have been reported less frequently than porphyria.

HCB is a mixed-type cytochrome-P-450-inducing compound, with phenobarbital-inducible and 3-methylcholanthrene-inducible properties. It is known to bind to the Ah receptor.

In chronic studies, mild effects on the liver (histopathological changes, enzyme induction) occurred in several studies of rats exposed to between 0.25 and 0.6 mg HCB/kg body weight per day; the NOELs in these studies were 0.05 to 0.07 mg HCB/kg body weight per day. Concentrations of neurotransmitters in the hypothalamus were altered in mink dams with chronic dietary exposure to 0.16 mg HCB/kg body weight per day, and in their offspring exposed throughout gestation and nursing. Calcium homoeostasis and bone morphometry were affected in subchronic studies on rats at 0.7 mg HCB/kg body weight per day, but not at 0.07 mg/kg body weight per day.

The carcinogenicity of HCB has been assessed in several adequate bioassays on rodents. In hamsters fed diets yielding average doses of 4, 8 or 16 mg/kg body weight per day for life, there were increases in the incidence of liver cell tumours (hepatomas) in both sexes at all doses, haemangioendotheliomas of the liver at 8-16 mg/kg body weight per day, and adenomas of the thyroid in males at the highest dose. Dietary exposure of mice to 6, 12 and 24 mg/kg body weight per day for 120 weeks resulted in an increase in the incidence of liver cell tumours (hepatomas) in both sexes at the two higher doses (not significant, except for females at the highest dose). *In utero*, lactational and oral exposure of rats to HCB in diets yielding average lifetime doses ranging from 0.01 to 1.5 mg/kg body weight per day (males) or 1.9 mg/kg body weight per day (females) for up to 130 weeks *post utero* produced increased incidences, at the highest dose, of neoplastic liver nodules and adrenal phaeochromocytomas in females and of parathyroid adenomas in males. In another long-term study on rats, exposure for up to 2 years to diets yielding average HCB doses of 4-5 and 8-9 mg/kg body weight per day induced increases in the incidences of hepatomas and of renal cell adenomas at both doses in both sexes, and of hepatocellular carcinomas, bile duct adenomas/carcinomas and adrenal phaeochromocytomas and adrenal cortical adenomas in females. High incidences of liver tumours have also been reported in some more limited studies in which single dietary concentrations were administered to small groups of female rats. In addition, it has been reported that, following subchronic dietary exposure to HCB, mice, hamsters and rats developed tumours in the liver, bile duct, kidney, thymus, spleen and lymph nodes. Dietary exposure to HCB promoted the induction of liver tumours by polychlorinated terphenyl in mice and by diethylnitrosamine in rats.

Except in the case of renal tumours in male rats (which appear at least in part to be the result of hyaline droplet nephropathy) and hepatomas in rats (which may result from hyperplastic responses to hepatocellular necrosis), mechanistic studies that address the relevance to humans of the tumour types induced by HCB have not been identified.

HCB has little capability to induce directly gene mutation, chromosomal damage and DNA repair. It exhibited weak mutagenic activity in a small number of the available studies on bacteria and yeast, although it should be noted that each of these studies has limitations. There is also some evidence of low-level binding to DNA *in vitro* and *in vivo*, but at levels well below those expected for genotoxic carcinogens.

In studies of reproduction, oral exposure of monkeys to as little as 0.1 mg HCB/kg body weight per day for 90 days affected the light microscopic structure and ultrastructure of the surface germinal epithelium, an unusual target for ovarian toxins. This dose also caused ultrastructural injury to the primordial germ cells. These specific target sites, which are damaged further at higher doses, were associated with otherwise normal follicular, oocyte and embryo development, suggesting specificity of HCB action within the site of the ovary. Male reproduction was only affected at much higher doses (between 30 and 221 mg/kg body weight per day) in studies on several non-primate species.

Transplacental or lactational exposure of rats and cats to maternal doses of between 3 and 4 mg/kg body weight per day was found to be hepatotoxic and/or affected the survival or growth of nursing offspring. In some cases, these or higher doses reduced litter sizes and/or increased the number of stillbirths. (Adverse effects on suckling infants have generally been observed more frequently, and at lower doses, than embryotoxic or fetotoxic effects). The offspring of mink with chronic exposure to as little as 1 mg HCB/kg diet (approximately 0.16 mg/kg body weight per day) had reduced birth weight and increased mortality to weaning. Although skeletal and renal abnormalities have been observed in fetuses in some studies of rats and mice exposed to HCB during gestation, these were either not clearly related to treatment or occurred at doses that were also maternally toxic. In two studies, one of which included lactational and postnatal exposure, neurobehavioural development of rat pups was affected by *in utero* exposure to HCB at oral maternal doses of 0.64 to 2.5 mg HCB/kg body weight per day.

The results of a number of studies have indicated that HCB affects the immune system. Rats or monkeys exposed to between 3 and 120 mg HCB/kg body weight per day had histopathological alterations in the thymus, spleen, lymph nodes and/or lymphoid tissues of the lung. Chronic exposure of beagle dogs to 0.12 mg/kg body weight per day caused nodular hyperplasia of the gastric lymphoid tissue. In a number of studies on rats, humoral immunity and, to a lesser extent, cell-mediated immunity were enhanced by several weeks exposure to HCB in the diet, while macrophage function was unaltered. As little as 4 mg HCB/kg diet (approximately 0.2 mg/kg body weight per day) during gestation, through nursing and to 5 weeks of age increased humoral and cell-mediated immune responses and caused accumulation of macrophages in the lung tissue of rat pups. In contrast, HCB has been found to be immunosuppressive in most studies with mice; doses of as little as 0.5-0.6 mg/kg body weight per day for several weeks depressed resistance to infection by *Leishmania* or to a challenge with tumour cells, decreased cytotoxic macrophage activity of the spleen, and reduced the delayed-type hypersensitivity response in offspring exposed *in utero* and through nursing. In a number of studies on various strains of rats, short-term or subchronic exposure to HCB affected thyroid function, as indicated by decreased serum levels of total and free thyroxine (T_4) and often, to a lesser extent, triiodothyronine (T_3).

1.7 Effects on humans

Most data on the effects of HCB on humans originate from accidental poisonings that took place in Turkey in 1955-1959, in which more than 600 cases of porphyria cutanea tarda (PCT) were identified. In this incident, disturbances in porphyrin metabolism, dermatological lesions, hyperpigmentation, hypertrichosis, enlarged liver, enlargement of the thyroid gland and lymph nodes, and (in roughly half the cases) osteoporosis or arthritis were observed, primarily in children. Breast-fed infants of mothers exposed to HCB in this incident developed a disorder called pembe yara (pink sore), and most died within a year. There is also limited evidence that PCT occurs in humans with relatively high exposure to HCB in the workplace or in the general environment.

The few available epidemiological studies of cancer are limited by small size, poorly characterized exposures to HCB and exposure to numerous other agents, and are insufficient to assess the carcinogenicity of HCB to humans.

1.8 Effects on other organisms in the laboratory and field

In studies of the acute toxicity of HCB to aquatic organisms, exposure to concentrations in the range of 1 to 17 µg/litre reduced production of chlorophyll in algae and reproduction in ciliate protozoa, and caused mortality in pink shrimp and grass shrimp, but did not cause mortality in freshwater or marine fish. In longer-term studies, the growth of sensitive freshwater algae and protozoa was affected by a concentration of 1 µg/litre, while concentrations of approximately 3 µg/litre caused mortality in amphipods and liver necrosis in large-mouth bass.

1.9 Evaluation of human health risks and effects on the environment

1.9.1 Health effects

The Task Group concluded that the available data are sufficient to develop guidance values for non-neoplastic and neoplastic effects of HCB.

For non-neoplastic effects, based on the lowest reported NOEL (0.05 mg HCB/kg body weight per day), for primarily hepatic effects observed at higher doses in studies on pigs and rats exposed by the oral route, and incorporating an uncertainty factor of 300 (x 10 for interspecies variation, x 10 for intraspecies variation, and x 3 for severity of effect), a TDI of 0.17 µg/kg body weight per day has been derived.

The approach for neoplastic effects is based on the tumorigenic dose TD_5 i.e., the intake associated with a 5% excess incidence of tumours in experimental studies in animals. Based on the results of the two-generation carcinogenicity bioassay in rats and using the multi-stage model, the TD_5 value is 0.81 mg/kg body weight per day for neoplastic nodules of the liver in females. Based on consideration of the insufficient mechanistic data, an uncertainty factor of 5000 was used to develop a health-based guidance value of 0.16 µg/kg body weight per day.

1.9.2 Environmental effects

The Task Group pointed out that there are very few experimental studies on which an environmental risk assessment can be made. Levels of HCB in surface water are generally several orders lower than those expected to present a hazard to aquatic organisms, except in a few extremely contaminated locations. However, HCB concentrations in the eggs of sea birds and raptors from a number of locations from around the world approach those associated with reduced embryo weights in herring gulls (1500 µg/kg), suggesting that HCB has the potential to harm embryos of sensitive bird species. Similarly, levels of HCB in fish at a number of sites worldwide are within an order of magnitude of the dietary level of 1000 µg/kg associated with reduced birth weight and increased mortality of offspring in mink. This suggests that HCB has the potential to cause adverse effects in mink and perhaps other fish-eating mammals.

1.10 Conclusions

a) HCB is a persistent chemical that bioaccumulates owing to its lipid solubility and resistance to breakdown.

b) Animal studies have shown that HCB causes cancer and affects a wide range of organ systems including the liver, lungs, kidneys, thyroid, reproductive tissues and nervous and immune systems.

c) Clinical toxicity, including porphyria cutanea tarda in children and adults, and mortality in nursing infants, has been observed in humans with high accidental exposure.

d) Various measures are warranted to reduce the environmental burden of HCB.

e) The following health-based guidance values for the total daily intake (TDI) of HCB in humans have been suggested: for non-cancer effects, 0.17 μg/kg body weight/day; for neoplastic effects, 0.16 μg/kg body weight/day.

2. IDENTITY, PHYSICAL AND CHEMICAL PROPERTIES, AND ANALYTICAL METHODS

2.1 Identity

Hexachlorobenzene (HCB) is a chlorinated aromatic hydrocarbon with the chemical formula C_6Cl_6. Its CAS registry number is 118-74-1.

Structure:

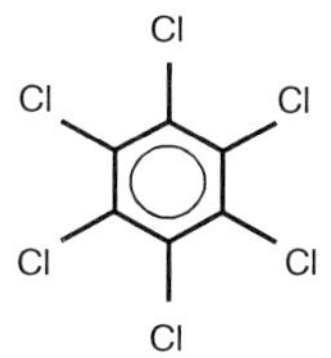

Synonyms: perchlorobenzene, pentachlorophenyl chloride, phenyl perchloryl

Trade names: Amatin, Anticarie, Bunt Cure, Bunt-No-More, Co-op Hexa, Granox NM, Julin's Carbon Chloride, No Bunt, No Bunt 40, No Bunt 80, No Bunt Liquid, Sanocide, Smut-Go, Snieciotox, HexaCB

2.2 Physical and chemical properties

Some physical and chemical properties of HCB are listed in Table 1. At ambient temperature, HCB is a white crystalline that is virtually insoluble in water, but is soluble in ether, benzene and chloroform (NTP, 1994). It has a high octanol/water partition coefficient, low vapour pressure, moderate Henry's Law constant and low flammability. Technical grade HCB is available as a wettable powder, liquid and dust (NTP, 1994). Technical grade HCB contains about 98% HCB, 1.8% pentachlorobenzene and 0.2% 1,2,4,5-tetrachlorobenzene (IARC, 1979), and it is known to contain a variety of impurities, including hepta- and octachlorodibenzofurans, octachlorodibenzo-*p*-dioxin and decachlorobiphenyl (Villanueva et al., 1974; Goldstein et al., 1978).

Table 1. Physical and chemical properties of hexachlorobenzene[a]

Property	Value
Relative molecular mass	284.79
Melting point (°C)	230
Boiling point (°C)	322 (sublimates)
Density (g/cm^3 at 20 °C)	1.5691
Vapour pressure (Pa at 25 °C)	0.0023
Log octanol/water partition coefficient	5.5
Water solubility (mg/litre at 25 °C)	0.005
Henry's Law Constant (calculated)[b] (Pa/mol per m^3)	131
Conversion factors	1 ppm = 11.8 mg/m^3 1 mg/m^3 = 0.08 ppm

[a] From ATSDR (1990); Mackay et al. (1992)
[b] The Henry's Law Constant has been calculated using the tabled values for aqueous solubility and vapour pressure

2.3 Analytical methods

Analytical methods for the determination of HCB in environmental samples and biological tissues vary depending upon the matrix and representative methods for various matrices, and are summarized in Tables 2 and 3.

Table 2. Analytical methods for determining hexachlorobenzene in environmental samples[a]

Sample matrix	Sample preparation	Analytical method[b]	Sample detection limit	Recovery	Reference
Water	Extract with dichloromethane, exchange to hexane, concentrate; Florisil column chromatography as a clean-up	GC/ECD	0.05 mg/kg	95 ± 10-20%	US EPA (1982)
Water	Extract with dichloromethane at pH 11 and 2, concentrate	GC/MS	1.9 mg/kg	No data	US EPA (1982)
Air	Glass fibre filter and XAD2 traps separated by a PUF disk; extraction with toluene	HRGC/ LRMS	0.18 pg/m^3	>99%	Hippelein et al. (1993)
Air	Polyurethane foam (PUF) sampling cartridge, extraction with diethyl ether in hexane	GC/ECD	<0.1 µg/m^3	94.5±8%	Lewis & MacLeod (1982)
Air	Polyurethane foam (PUF) plugs, extraction with hexane, fractionation by HPLC	GC/ECD	low pg/m^3 range (not specified)	93±1.1%	Oehme & Stray (1982)

Table 2 (contd).

Sample matrix	Sample preparation	Analytical method[b]	Sample detection limit	Recovery	Reference
Air	Porous polyurethane foam (PUF), or Tenax-GC resin; filters refluxed with dichloro-methane and chlorinated solvents removed and refluxed with hexane; clean-up by alumina chromatography	GC/ECD	No data	Tenax more effective than PUF in retaining HCB	Billings & Bidleman (1980)
Air	Adsorb on Amberlite XAD-2 resin separated by a silanized glass wool plug, desorption with carbon tetrachloride.	GC/PID	0.014 mg/m^3	~95 ± 12%	Langhorst & Nestrick (1979)
Air	Trace Atmospheric Gas Analyser using negative atmospheric pressure chemical ionization for trace gas analysis; collection from ambient air and transfer into a carrier of CO_2 for analysis		~0.35 $\mu g/m^3$	No data	Thomson et al. (1980)

Table 2 (contd).

Soil, chemical waste disposal site samples	Hexane extraction	GC/ECD	10 mg/kg	78±2.6% to 96.5±3.6%	DeLeon et al. (1980)
Soil	Extract with dichloromethane	GC/MS	18 mg/kg 5 mg/kg	No data	US EPA (1986b)
Sediment	Solvent extraction subjected to acid-base fractionation; base/neutral fraction subjected to silica gel chromatography	GC/MS		46%	Lopez-Avila et al. (1983)
Wastes, non-water miscible	Extract with dichloromethane	GC/MS	190 mg/kg 50 mg/kg	No data	US EPA (1986b)
Wastes, soil	Extract with dichloromethane	GC/MS	20 µg/litre[c]	No data	US EPA (1986b)

[a] Portions of the table were taken from ATSDR (1990)
[b] GC = gas chromatography; ECD = electron capture detector; MS = mass spectrometry; PID = photoionization detector; HRGC = high-resolution gas chromatography; LRMS = low-resolution mass spectrometry
[c] Identification limit; detection limits for actual samples are several orders of magnitude higher depending upon the sample matrix and extraction procedure employed.

Table 3. Analytical methods for determining hexachlorobenzene in biological materials

Sample matrix	Sample preparation	Analytical method	Sample detection limit	Recovery	Reference
Fish tissue	Grind with sodium sulfate, extract with hexane/acetone, clean-up by Na_2SO_4/ alumina/silica gel/Florisil column followed by a H_2SO_4 column on silica gel	GC/ECD	~0.05 µg/kg	No data	Oliver & Nicol (1982)
Fish tissue	Extraction with hexane/ isopropanol, solvent and sulfuric acid partitioning	GC/ECD	No data	No data	Lunde & Ofstad (1976)
Fish tissue	Sulfuric acid digestion, silica gel column chromatography, methylation, alumina column chromatography	GC/ECD	10-15 µg/kg	93%	Lamparski et al. (1980)
Oyster tissue	Extraction with acetone/acetonitrile, partitioning into petroleum ether, silica gel chromatography	GC/ECD	No data	No data	Murray et al. (1980)
Adipose tissue (chicken)	Extraction with hexane, subjected to Florisil clean-up and one-fraction elution	GC/ECD	No data	87.4-92.6%	Watts et al. (1980)
Adipose tissue	Extraction (solvent not specified), bulk lipid removal, Florisil fractionation	HRGC/MS	12 µg/kg	No data	Stanley (1986)
Adipose tissue	Extraction with benzene/acetone, Florisil fractionation	GC/ECD	0.12 µg/kg	79-95%	Mes (1992)

Table 3 (contd).

Blood/urine	Extraction with carbon tetrachloride, silica gel column chromatography, concentrate	GC/PID	4.1 µg/kg (urine) 16 µg/kg (blood)	83%	Langhorst & Nestrick (1979)
Blood	Extraction with hexane, concentrate	GC/ECD	No data	No data	US EPA (1980)
Blood	Extraction with hexane/isopropanol	GC/ECD	No data	No data	Lunde & Bjorseth (1977)
Breast milk	Extraction with acetone/benzene, Florisil fractionation	GC/ECD	33 µg/kg	70-82%	Mes et al. (1993)

GC = gas chromatography; ECD = electron capture detector; PID = photoionization detector; HRGC = high-resolution gas chromatography; MS = mass spectrometry

3. SOURCES OF HUMAN AND ENVIRONMENTAL EXPOSURE

3.1 Sources, uses and production processes

Industrial synthesis of HCB may be achieved through the chlorination of benzene at 150-200 °C using a ferric chloride catalyst or from the distillation of residues from the production of tetrachloroethylene (US EPA, 1985a). HCB may also be synthesized by refluxing hexachlorocyclohexane isomers with sulfuryl chloride or chlorosulfonic acid in the presence of a ferric chloride or aluminum catalyst (Brooks & Hunt, 1984).

Historically, HCB had many uses in industry and agriculture. The major agricultural application for HCB used to be as a seed dressing for crops such as wheat, barley, oats and rye to prevent growth of fungi. The use of HCB in such applications was discontinued in many countries in the 1970s owing to concerns about adverse effects on the environment and human health. HCB may continue to be used for this purpose in some countries; for example, HCB was still used in 1986 as a fungicide, seed-dressing and scabicide in sheep in Tunisia (Jemaa et al., 1986). However, it is uncertain as to whether HCB is still used for this purpose.

In industry, HCB has been used directly in the manufacture of pyrotechnics, tracer bullets and as a fluxing agent in the manufacture of aluminum. HCB has also been used as a wood-preserving agent, a porosity-control agent in the manufacture of graphite anodes, and as a peptizing agent in the production of nitroso and styrene rubber for tyres (Mumma & Lawless, 1975). It is likely that some of these applications have been discontinued, although no information is available.

Although HCB production has ceased in most countries, it is still being generated inadvertently as a by-product and/or impurity in several chemical processes. HCB is formed as a reaction by-product of thermal chlorination, oxychlorination, and pyrolysis operations in the manufacture of chlorinated solvents (mainly carbon tetrachloride, trichloroethylene and tetrachloroethylene) (Government of Canada, 1993). The concentrations of HCB in distillation bottoms was estimated to be 25%, 15% and 5%, respectively, for tetrachloroethylene, carbon tetrachloride and trichloroethylene (Jacoff et al., 1986). While HCB could potentially also be a contaminant in the final product, it was not detected (detection limit 5 mg/litre) in carbon tetrachloride and tetrachloroethylene in an investigation in Canada (personal communication to Health Canada by Mr John Schultiess, Dow Chemical Canada Inc., 1991). Analysis of production lots of tri- and tetrachloroethylene produced in Europe in 1996 failed to detect HCB at a detection limit of 2 µg/litre solvent (personal communication to the IPCS by Mr C. de Rooij, Solvay Corporation Europe, 1996).

HCB is also generated as a waste by-product during the manufacture of chlorinated solvents, chlorinated aromatics and pesticides (Jacoff et al., 1986). The waste streams from the production of pentachloronitrobenzene (PCNB), chlorothalonil and dacthal are expected to contribute the bulk of HCB released from the pesticide industry (Brooks & Hunt, 1984), although HCB can also be generated as a waste by-product from the production of pentachlorophenol, atrazine, simazine, propazine and maleic hydrazide (Quinlivan et al., 1975; Mumma & Lawless, 1975). These pesticides are also known to contain HCB as an impurity in the final product, usually at levels of less than 1% HCB when appropriate procedures are used for the synthesis and purification stages (Tobin, 1986). When such procedures are not met, the level of HCB could be much higher (e.g., pentachloronitrobenzene has been reported to contain 1.8-11% HCB (Tobin, 1986)). However, owing to many voluntary and regulatory pressures, it is unlikely that such high levels of HCB are present in today's pesticide formulations, but no information is available to substantiate this point.

The chlor-alkali industry produces chlorine (Cl_2), hydrogen and caustic soda ($NaOH$) by electrolysis of purified and concentrated sodium chloride ($NaCl$). Processes using graphite anodes are known to produce HCB as a by-product (Quinlivan et al., 1975; Mumma & Lawless, 1975; Alves & Chevalier, 1980) owing to the reaction of chlorine with graphite anode materials such as carbon and oils. Depending on the purification procedures, the final products might also be contaminated with HCB. In some countries, graphite anodes have been replaced by dimensionally stabilized anodes (DSA), which do not generate HCB (Government of Canada, 1993).

Incineration is an important source of HCB in the environment. Emission levels from incinerators are very site-specific, and therefore generic levels are difficult to estimate. Earlier information yielded a crude estimate of the total HCB released from all municipal incinerators in the USA to be 57-454 kg/year (US EPA, 1986a), but levels currently emitted are not known.

3.2 World production levels

Few recent data on the quantities of HCB produced are available. Worldwide production of pure HCB was estimated to be 10 000 tonnes/year for the years 1978-1981 (Rippen & Frank, 1986). An estimated 300 tonnes was produced by three manufacturers in the USA in 1973 (IARC, 1979). HCB was produced/imported in the European Community at 8000 tonnes/year in 1978 (Rippen & Frank, 1986), and a company in Spain used to produce an estimated 150 tonnes of HCB annually (IARC, 1979). Approximately 1500 tonnes of HCB were manufactured annually in Germany for the production of the rubber auxiliary PCTP (BUA, 1994), but this production was discontinued in 1993. No further centres of HCB manufacture in Europe or North America have been identified. Production of HCB has declined as a result of restrictions on its use starting in the 1970s.

Considerable amounts of HCB are inadvertently produced as a by-product in the manufacture of chlorinated solvents, chlorinated aromatics and chlorinated pesticides. Jacoff et al. (1986) estimated that approximately 4130 tonnes of HCB are generated annually as a waste product in the USA and that nearly 77% of this is produced from the manufacture of three chlorinated solvents: carbon tetrachloride, trichloroethylene and tetrachloroethylene. The remainder is produced by the chlorinated pesticide industry. In 1977, about 300 tonnes of HCB were generated in Japan as a waste by-product in the production of tetrachloroethylene, almost all of which was incinerated (IARC, 1979). It was estimated that >5000 tonnes HCB/year were produced as a by-product during tetrachloroethylene production in the Federal Republic of Germany in 1980 (Rippen & Frank, 1986). However, recent estimates for Europe from ECSA (European Chlorinated Solvent Association; P.G. Johnson (1996) personal communication to IPCS) indicate that up to 4000 tonnes/year of HCB are produced as a by-product during certain tetrachloroethylene production processes and that over 99% of this by-product was incinerated at high temperatures.

3.3 Entry into the environment

Currently, the principal sources of HCB in the environment are estimated to be the manufacture of chlorinated solvents, the manufacture and application of HCB-contaminated pesticides, and inadequate incineration of chlorine-containing wastes. It should be noted that only a small fraction of the HCB generated as a by-product may be released, depending on the process technology and waste-disposal practices employed. For example, according to the US Toxic Chemical Release Inventory (TRI), releases of HCB from the ten largest processing facilities were 460 kg, most of this to air, compared with almost 542 000 kg transferred offsite as waste. The TRI data are not comprehensive, since only certain types of facilities are required to report (ATSDR, 1994). ECSA (P.G. Johnson, personal communication to IPCS) estimated that European emissions of HCB were about 200 kg/year in 1993.

As discussed in the previous section, HCB is a contaminant of a number of chlorinated pesticides. Since most current applications for these products are dispersive, most HCB from this source will be released to the environment.

Substantial quantities of HCB are also contained in the wastes generated through the manufacture of chlorinated solvents and pesticides. In the mid-1980s in the USA, 81% of these HCB-containing wastes were disposed of by incineration, compared to 19% via landfilling (Jacoff et al., 1986). It is likely that the amount of HCB wastes disposed of by incineration has since increased, although information has not been found to confirm this point. HCB can be emitted from incinerators as a result of incomplete thermal decomposition of these wastes and as a product of incomplete combustion (PIC) from the thermal decomposition of a variety of chlorinated organics such as Kepone, mirex, chlorobenzenes, polychlorinated biphenyls, pentachlorophenol, polyvinyl chloride and mixtures of chlorinated solvents (Ahling et al., 1978; Dellinger et al., 1991).

Although only a small proportion of the HCB-containing waste generated in the USA is landfilled, HCB may continue to leach to groundwater from previously landfilled HCB waste sites. The contribution of this route is uncertain, although HCB is not easily leached, and landfills containing HCB are now designed to prevent leachate losses into adjacent water systems (Brooks & Hunt, 1984). HCB emission into the atmosphere from landfills containing HCB wastes occurs from slow volatilization and from displacement of the contaminated soil (Brooks & Hunt, 1984).

HCB has been detected in emissions from a number of industries, including paint manufacturers, coal and steel producers, pulp and paper mills, textile mills, pyrotechnics producers, aluminum smelters, soap producers and wood-preservation facilities (Quinlivan et al., 1975; Gilbertson, 1979; Alves & Chevalier, 1980), probably reflecting the use of products contaminated with HCB. Municipal and industrial wastewater facilities may also discharge HCB-contaminated effluents (Environment Canada/Ontario Ministry of the Environment, 1986; King & Sherbin, 1986), probably owing to inputs from industrial sources.

Long-range transport plays a significant role as a means of redistribution of HCB throughout the environment. Wet deposition (deposition via rain or snowfall) is the primary mechanism for transport of HCB from the atmosphere to aquatic and terrestrial systems in Canada (Eisenreich & Strachan, 1992). For example, it is estimated that long-range transport and total deposition to the Canadian environment is approximately 510 kg/year, an amount that is similar to that from all other sources combined (Government of Canada, 1993).

4. ENVIRONMENTAL TRANSPORT, DISTRIBUTION AND TRANSFORMATION

4.1 Environmental transport and degradation

HCB is distributed throughout the environment because it is mobile and resistant to degradation. Volatilization from water to air and sedimentation following adsorption to suspended particulates are the major removal processes from water (Oliver, 1984a; Oliver & Charlton, 1984). Once in the sediments, HCB will tend to accumulate and become trapped by overlying sediments (Oliver & Nicol, 1982). Although HCB is not readily leached from soils and sediments, some desorption does occur and may be a continuous source of HCB to the environment, even if inputs to the system cease (Oliver, 1984a; Oliver et al., 1989). Chemical or biological degradation is not considered to be important for the removal of HCB from water or sediments (Callahan et al., 1979; Mansour et al., 1986; Mill & Haag, 1986; Oliver & Carey, 1986). In the troposphere, HCB is transported over long distances by virtue of its persistence, but does undergo slow photolytic degradation (the half-life is approximately 80 days; Mill & Haag, 1986), or is removed from the air phase via atmospheric deposition to water and soil (Bidleman et al., 1986; Ballschmiter & Wittlinger, 1991; Lane et al., 1992a, 1992b). In soil, volatilization is the major removal process at the surface (Kilzer et al., 1979; Griffin & Chou, 1981; Schwarzenbach et al., 1983; Nash & Gish, 1989), while slow aerobic (half-life of 2.7-5.7 years) and anaerobic biodegradation (half-life of 10.6-22.9 years) are the major removal processes at lower depths (Beck & Hansen, 1974; Howard et al., 1991).

4.2 Bioaccumulation and biomagnification

The bioaccumulative properties of HCB result from the combination of its physicochemical properties (high octanol/water partition coefficient) and its slow elimination due to limited metabolism related to its high chemical stability. Organisms generally accumulate HCB from water and from food, although benthic organisms may also accumulate HCB directly from sediment (Oliver, 1984b; Knezovich & Harrison, 1988; Gobas et al., 1989). The uptake of HCB in benthic invertebrates has been investigated in a number of laboratory and field studies. The results demonstrated that some HCB in sediments is available to infaunal species. Reported bioaccumulation factors[a] (BAF) for invertebrates in HCB-containing sediments range from 0.04 to 0.58 in high-organic-content sediment to 1.95 in low-organic-content sediment (Oliver, 1984b; Knezovich & Harrison, 1988; Gobas et al., 1989). The bioavailability of sediment-bound HCB is inversely related to sediment organic carbon content (Knezovich & Harrison, 1988), and varies with the type and size of the organisms and their feeding habits (Boese et al., 1990), the extent of contact with sediment pore and interstitial waters (Landrum, 1989), and the surface area of the substrate (Swindoll & Applehans, 1987). Landrum (1989) suggested that the bioavailability of sediment-sorbed chemicals declines as the contact time between the sediment and a contaminant increases. For example, Schuytema et al., (1990) observed that addition of HCB-spiked sediments did not result in a significant increase in the uptake of HCB by the worm (*Lumbriculus variegatus*), amphipods (*Hyalella azteca* and *Gammarus lacustris*), and fathead minnows (*Pimephales promelas*) in a laboratory recirculating water/sediment system. However, there was a substantial increase of HCB levels in bed sediment, suggesting that sediment served as a more effective sink for HCB than the organisms.

The biomagnification factor (BMF) for HCB in the earthworm *Eisenia andrei* after exposure via food was 0.068 on a wet weight basis (0.071 on a lipid basis) (Belfroid et al., 1994a), the biota lipid-to-soil accumulation factor, defined as the ratio of the concentration in the animal to that on the soil, was 215 g soil dry weight/g lipid (Belfroid et al., 1994b), and the bioconcentration factors (BCFs) for earthworms kept in water were found to be between 48 x 10^4 and 62 x 10^4 ml water/g lipid (Belfroid et al., 1993).

Field studies indicate that exposure via food is important for organisms at higher trophic levels, as significant biomagnification has been observed in several studies in natural aquatic ecosystems. In Lake Ontario, Oliver & Niimi (1988) observed that tissue residue concentrations increased from plankton (mean = 1.6 ng/g wet weight)

---

[a] Defined as tissue concentration (wet weight) divided by sediment concentration (dry weight). BAFs from Oliver (1984b) were divided by 6.67 to convert tissue dry weight to wet weight.

to mysids (mean = 4.0 ng/g wet weight) to alewives (mean = 20 ng/g wet weight) to salmonids (mean = 38 ng/g wet weight). Braune & Norstrom (1989) used field data on body burdens of HCB in the herring gull (*Larus argentatus*) and one of its principal food items, the alewife (*Alosa pseudoharengus*) in a Great Lakes food chain to calculate a biomagnification factor (whole body, wet weight basis) of 31.

5. ENVIRONMENTAL LEVELS AND HUMAN EXPOSURE

5.1 Environmental levels

HCB has been detected in air, water, sediment, soil and biota. Representative levels reported in various environmental media in many countries are presented in Tables 4, 5 and 6.

5.1.1 Air

HCB is widely dispersed in ambient air, and is generally present at low concentrations. Mean concentrations of HCB in air removed from point sources in Canada, Norway, Sweden, Germany, the USA, the Arctic and the Antarctic range from 0.04 to 0.6 ng/m^3 (Table 4). Levels of HCB in air are generally similar between urban, rural and remote sites, reflecting the persistence and long-range transport of this substance.

Airborne concentrations of HCB measured in the USA near nine chlorinated solvent and pesticide plants in 1973 and 1976 were much higher than background levels (Spigarelli et al., 1986). Concentrations as high as 24 μg/m^3 were detected in the immediate vicinity of one plant, while the maximum concentration of HCB distant from the site was 0.36 μg/m^3. The highest levels were associated with the production of perchloroethylene, trichloroethylene and carbon tetrachloride, and with plants where onsite landfill and open pit waste disposal were practiced. More recently, Grimalt et al. (1994) reported that airborne concentrations of HCB in a community in the vicinity of a organochlorine factory built in 1898 in Catalonia, Spain, averaged 35 ng/m^3, compared with 0.3 ng/m^3 in Barcelona, the reference community for this study. It is not known how representative the data from these studies are, as HCB releases are expected to be minimized from industries using appropriate modern technology and waste management practices.

No data are available on the levels of HCB in indoor air.

Table 4. Levels of hexachlorobenzene in ambient air (ng/m^3)

Location	Year	Detection limit	Mean	Range[a]	Reference
Canada (Windsor, Ontario)	1987-1990	0.03	0.13	ND-0.44	Environment Canada (1992)
Canada (Ontario)					
- industrial/urban areas	1985-1989	0.007	0.167	0.07-0.31	Lane et al. (1992b)
- rural areas			0.094	0.02-0.31	
Canada (Egbert, Ontario)	1988-1989	-	>0.054	0.00004-0.64	Hoff et al. (1992)
Canada (Walpole Island)	1988-1989	0.02	0.15	ND-0.34	Environment Canada (1992)
Canadian High Arctic (Beaufort Sea)	1987		0.15	ND-0.154	Patton et al. (1989)
Bear Island (Arctic)					Oehme & Stray (1982)
- summer		0.001	0.04	0.029-0.045	
- winter		0.001	0.111	0.059-0.188	
Southern Ocean and Antarctica	1990		0.06	0.04-0.078	Bidleman et al. (1993)
Enewetak Atoll (Pacific Ocean)	1979		0.10	0.095-0.13	Atlas & Giam (1981)

Table 4 (contd).

Location	Year	Detection limit	Mean	Range[a]	Reference
Spitzbergen					
- summer		0.001	0.071	0.05-0.085	Oehme & Stray (1982)
- winter		0.001	0.086	0.071-0.095	
Germany (Hamburg - residential, suburban and industrial sites)	1986-1987		0.6	0.3-2.5	Bruckmann et al. (1988)
South Germany	1986-1990		0.21	0.058-0.52	Morosini et al. (1993)
Norway (Lillestrom)		0.001	0.162	0.055-0.234	Oehme & Stray (1982)
Sweden (Aspvreten)	1984		0.067	0.054->0.165	Bidleman et al. (1987)
Sweden (Stockholm)	1983-1985		0.07	0.054->0.130	Bidleman et al. (1987)
Spain - (near organochlorine compounds factory)	1989 & 1992	-	35	11-44	Grimalt et al. (1994)
- hospital in Barcelona		-	0.3	0.25-0.4	

Table 4 (contd).

USA (Portland, Oregon)	1984		0.075	0.05-0.11	Ligocki et al. (1985)
USA - chemical production plants				ND-24000	Spigarelli et al. (1986)
USA - urban areas	1975-1979	0.1	0.5	ND-4.4	Carey et al. (1985)

[a] ND = not detected

5.1.2 Water

Levels of HCB in freshwater in Europe and North America are generally below 1 ng/litre (Table 5), although higher values have been reported in aquatic systems that receive industrial discharges and surface run-off. In the connecting channels to the Great Lakes in Canada, HCB levels were often found to exceed 1.0 ng/litre, particularly near point sources. Levels in the St. Clair River near the Dow Chemical outfall were as high as 87 ng/litre in 1985 and 75 ng/litre in 1986 (Oliver & Kaiser, 1986).

Mean concentrations of HCB in seawater rarely exceed 1 ng/litre (Table 5) (Ernst, 1986; Burton & Bennett, 1987). In the Nueces Estuary in Texas, USA, the highest level (0.61 ng/litre) was found near sewage outfalls (Ray et al., 1983a). Higher concentrations (up to 196 ng/litre) were observed in the Forth Estuary in Scotland, near domestic and chemical industry discharges (Rogers et al., 1989).

5.1.3 Soil

Data identified on levels of HCB in soil are quite limited and are summarized in Table 6. The most extensive data are from the 1972 US National Soils Monitoring Program, in which the concentrations of a variety of pesticides were determined at 1483 sites from 37 states (Carey et al., 1979). HCB was detected at 11 sites, with a range of concentrations in positive samples from 10 to 440 μg/kg dry weight. Of 24 samples of agricultural soil in British Columbia, Canada, where HCB had last been applied as a seed treatment 10-15 years prior to the survey, 6 had detectable HCB residues of between 1.3 and 2.2 ng/g dry weight (Wilson & Wan, 1982).

Mean concentrations of HCB reported from uncontaminated soil in Europe were found to range from 0.3 ng/g in Switzerland (Müller, 1982) to 5.1 ng/g in a Swedish rural heathland soil (Thomas et al., 1985) (it was not indicated whether concentrations were on a dry or wet weight basis). Soil from a farming area in Italy contained 40 ng/g (dry or wet weight basis not indicated) (Leoni & D'Arca, 1976). HCB levels were not markedly increased by long-term application of sludge to land in Germany at a rate of 50 to 500 tons per ha and averaged 2.8 ng/g (dry or wet weight basis not indicated) (Witte et al., 1988a,b). Monitoring programmes in Germany yielded average

Table 5. Concentrations of hexachlorobenzene (ng/litre) in drinking-water and surface water

Source	Year	Detection limit	Mean	Range	Reference
Drinking-water					
Canada (Ontario)	1980	0.01	0.1	0.06-0.2	Oliver & Nicol (1982)
Canada (Maritime Provinces)	1985-1988	2.0		ND	Environment Canada (1989)
Croatia					
- Sisak	1988-1989	0.5	1.0[a]	<1-4	Fingler et al. (1992)
- Zagreb			2.0[a]	1-3	
USA	1977-1981	100	ND		US EPA (1985b)
Surface water					
Canada					
- Lake Superior	1986	0.007	0.026	0.018-0.040	Stevens & Neilson (1989)
- Lake Huron			0.033	0.018-0.073	
- Georgian Bay			0.041	0.032-0.054	
- Lake Erie			0.078	0.025-0.260	
- Lake Ontario			0.063	0.020-0.113	
Canada-St. Clair River	1985			0.30-87	Oliver & Kaiser (1986)
- tributaries to St. Clair R.				0.08-0.79	

Table 5 (contd).

Source	Year	Detection limit	Mean	Range	Reference
Canada (Atlantic Region); lakes, streams, reservoirs, estuaries, coastal waters	1979-1989	2.0		ND-2.2	Leger 1991
Germany (Elbe)	1990	-	12	3-62	BUA (1994)
Greece (Strimon River)	1985-1986	-	1.52	0.5-2.8	Kilikidis *et al.* (1992)
Italy (tributaries to Adriatic Sea)	1977-1978	1.0		ND	Galassi & Provini (1981)
Mediterranean Sea	1982-1983	0.1	2.13	ND-12.6	El-Dib & Badawy (1985)
Netherlands/Belgium	1993	10	<10	<10	RIWA (1993)
Netherlands	1987	-	<10	ND-100	De Walle et al. (1995)
North Sea (coastal waters and estuaries)	1979-1980		2.7	0.03-15	Ernst (1986)
Scotland (Forth Estuary)	1987	0.01		<0.01-196	Rogers et al. (1989)
Scotland (Forth Estuary)	1990			0.7-8.0	Harper et al. (1992)

Table 5 (contd).

Spain (Ebre Delta)	1985-1986	0.0005	0.041	ND-1.0	Grimalt et al. (1988)
USA (Texas-estuary)	1980		0.24	<0.01-0.61	Ray et al. (1983a)
USA (coastal, surface microlayer)		<0.1		<0.1-26	Cross et al. (1987)

[a] median value

Table 6. Levels of hexachlorobenzene in soil (ng/g dry weight)

Source	Year	Detection limit	Mean	Range	Reference
Canada (British Columbia)		1.0			Wilson & Wan (1982)
- agricultural soils				<1.0-2.2	
- near a former grain treatment plant				260 ng/g	
Czech/Polish Border (Giant Mountains)	-	-	3.25	0.47-4.8	Holoubek et al. (1994)
Germany (contaminated soil)	1989			0.3-339	Hagenmaier et al. (1992)
India	1987		24[a]	0-165	Nair & Pillai (1989)
Italy (farming area)	1971-1972		40		Leoni & D'Arca (1976)
Netherlands - Ochten	1993	-	18	5.1-66	Hendriks et al. (1995)
- Gelderse Poort			80	73-89	
Netherlands	1987	-	<10	<80	De Walle et al. (1995)
Sweden			5.1		Thomas et al. (1985)
USA	1968-1973			10-440	Carey et al. (1979)

Table 6 (contd).

USA (chemical plants)		0.002		ND-5 700 000	Spigarelli et al. (1986)
USA (hazardous waste sites)	1977-1978			20 000-400 000	Davis & Morgan (1986)
USA (5 locations near Love Canal)		0.1	1.04-5.6	0.15-26.3	Ding et al. (1992)

[a] ng/g wet weight

levels of HCB contamination of soil ranging from approximately 1 ng/g dry weight in the North Rhine-Westphalia (1990) to approximately 6 ng/g dry weight in Baden-Württemberg (1988) (BUA, 1994).

Levels in soil are highest near industrial sources of HCB. Levels as high as 12 600 ng/g dry weight were reported at one landfill site in Canada (Wilson & Wan, 1982), and 570 µg/g (dry or wet weight not indicated) on the grounds of a chlorinated solvent and pesticide production plant in the USA (Spigarelli et al., 1986). Soils near a former grain treatment plant in Canada contained 260 ng/g dry weight of HCB (Wilson & Wan, 1982). Levels of HCB in soils from contaminated floodplains in the Netherlands ranged from 5.1 to 89 ng/g dry weight (Hendriks et al., 1995).

5.1.4 Sediment

HCB strongly sorbs to sediment and suspended matter, and differences in the concentrations in the water as well as in the composition of the sediments and suspended matter result in a wide range of concentrations in this medium.

In sediment samples collected from 1979 to 1989 in the Atlantic provinces of Canada, HCB was reported to be below the limit of detection of 0.2 ng/g dry weight in 140 of 152 samples (Leger, 1991). In surveys conducted from 1980 to 1983, HCB levels in sediments from the Great Lakes ranged from 0.02 to 840 ng/g dry weight (Oliver & Nicol, 1982; Fox et al., 1983; Kaminsky et al., 1983; Oliver & Bourbonniere, 1985; Bourbonniere et al., 1986; Oliver et al., 1989; IJC, 1989). Analyses of sediment cores from Lake Ontario indicated that levels of HCB have declined from the 1960s to the early 1980s but more recent data are not available to determine if this downward trend has continued (Oliver & Nicol, 1982; Oliver et al., 1989). HCB levels in sediment sampled from eight lakes in northern remote Canada (date of sampling not specified) ranged from 0.09 to 1.80 ng/g dry weight (Muir *et al.*, 1995).

Levels as high as 5100 ng/g dry weight were detected in the Rhine River in Baden-Württemberg, Germany, in 1986 (BUA, 1994). The majority of sediment samples taken from the rivers Rhine and Elbe between 1980 and 1990 contained levels of HCB between 10 and 500 ng/g dry weight, although levels below 1 ng/g dry weight were determined in some other locations (BUA, 1994). A Nordic study on chlorinated compounds in the Baltic, Kattegat and Skagerrak (Østfeldt et al., 1994) found HCB concentrations in sediment ranging from 1 to 20 ng/g loi (loss on ignition), the higher values occurring mainly in the Bothnian Bay. An extreme value of 63 ng/g loi was found in Öresund between Denmark and Sweden. Levels of HCB in sediment samples collected near effluent discharges along a stream in Pakistan ranged from <0.05 to 94.5 ng/g wet weight (Tehseen *et al.*, 1994).

Higher levels of HCB in sediments were reported in studies conducted near point sources. As much as 280 000 ng HCB/g dry weight was detected in 1985 downstream of the Dow Chemical sewer discharges in the St. Clair River, USA (Oliver & Pugsley, 1986).

5.1.5 Biota

HCB has been detected in invertebrates, fish, reptiles, birds and mammals from around the world. Following the detection of HCB in tissues of wild birds by De Vos in 1967, high residues were often found in predatory birds, whereas minor quantities were detected in fish, mussels and birds of the aquatic environment (Vos et al., 1968; Koeman et al., 1969). Based on Canadian data from monitoring studies in birds, HCB levels declined sharply from the mid-1970s (the earliest data available) and into the early 1980s, after which they levelled off (Noble & Elliott, 1986; Environment Canada/Department of Fisheries and Oceans/Health and Welfare Canada, 1991).

Levels of HCB in freshwater mussels in the Great Lakes and connecting channels have been found to range from 0.1 ng/g wet weight to 24 ng/g wet weight (Kauss & Hamdy, 1985; Innes et al., 1988; Muncaster et al., 1989). A similar range (4.4-26 ng/g wet weight) was observed in benthic amphipods, the pelagic amphipod *Pseudalibrotus litoralis* and brittle stars from the Beaufort Sea (Hargrave et al., 1989). Lower levels (0.1-1.8 ng/g wet weight) were observed in mussels (*Mytilus galloprovincialis*) from the Ebro Delta in the Western Mediterranean, and these levels were observed to decline from 1980 to 1992 (Solé et al., 1994). Levels in marine species of clams and oysters from the USA were reported in several studies to be < 1 ng/g wet weight (Phelps et al., 1986; Eisenberg & Topping, 1984; Ray et al., 1983b). Similarly, levels in invertebrates, including mussels (*Mytilus edulis*), soft clams (*Mya arenaria*), lugworms (*Arenicola marina*), and polychaetes (*Nereis diversicolor*), were

<1 ng/g fresh weight in the German Wadden Sea (Ernst, 1986). Bjerk & Brevik (1980) reported higher levels (50-350 ng/g wet weight) of HCB in crabs (*Carcinus maenas, Pagurus sp.*), snails (*Littorina littorea*), brittle stars (*Ophiura albida*) and sea stars (*Asteroidea*) from the contaminated Frierfjord in Norway, which receives discharge from various industries located in the region, and HCB and related compounds were reported to originate from one main source (unspecified) in the area. Østfeldt et al. (1994) found that mussels (*Mytilus edulis*) from the Baltic contain higher levels of HCB (200-800 ng/g lipid weight) than mussels from Kattegat (11-20 ng/g lipid weight).

In a 1981-1982 survey of HCB levels in fish from watersheds in Eastern Canada, whole body concentrations in brook trout (*Salvelinus fontinalis*) and yellow perch (*Perca flavescens*) ranged from below the limit of detection (4.2 ng/g in 1981; 0.2 ng/g in 1982) to 54 ng/g for trout and 15 ng/g wet weight for perch (Peterson & Ray, 1987). Relatively high body burdens of HCB have been observed in fish in Lake Ontario and connecting channels. HCB was not detected (ND) in juvenile spottail shiners (*Notropis hudsonius*) from Lakes Superior and Erie (detection level = 1 ng/g wet weight) (Suns et al., 1983; Environment Canada/Department of Fisheries and Oceans/Health and Welfare Canada, 1991), while mean body burdens in shiners in Lake Ontario ranged from ND to 13 ng/g wet weight, and those in the Detroit, Niagara, and St Clair rivers averaged 5 ng/g wet weight, ND to 8 ng/g wet weight, and 231 ng/g wet weight, respectively (Suns et al., 1985). Mean concentrations of HCB in the muscle tissue of various species of salmonids from Lake Ontario ranged from 5 to 37 ng/g wet weight (Niimi & Oliver, 1989).

Levels of HCB measured in whole fish species taken from major rivers and lakes in the USA (including known contaminated areas) ranged from <2 to 913 ng/g wet weight (Kuehl et al., 1983; DeVault, 1985; Schmitt et al., 1990; Kuehl & Butterworth, 1994). Levels in roach (*Rutilus rutilus L.*) and perch (*Perca fluviatilis L.*) from the "moderately polluted" Lahn River in Germany ranged from ND to 233 ng/g wet weight, with a mean of 1 ng/g (Schuler et al., 1985). Concentrations of HCB in the whole bodies of carp (*Cyprinus carpio*) from the mouth of tributaries to Lake Ontario and the Niagara River ranged from 52 to 1600 ng/g on a lipid basis (6.7 to 205 ng/g on a fresh weight basis). The highest values were measured near hazardous waste dumps and industrial facilities (as high as 1600 ng/g fat) (Jaffe

& Hites, 1986). Brunn & Manz (1982) reported a mean whole-body concentration of HCB in fish (mainly trout) from inland rivers, streams, and ponds in Germany of 5 ng/g wet weight. The highest levels were recorded from fish caught in rivers.

HCB levels in seawater are generally lower than those in freshwater, resulting in lower levels in edible parts of marine fish. In fish taken from the North Sea (species not reported), HCB levels in fish muscle tissues averaged 0.3-0.4 ng/g wet weight, with a maximum of 0.8 ng/g (Ernst, 1986). HCB concentrations in livers averaged 42 ng/g wet weight for cod (*Gadus morhua*) and 4 ng/g (range of 0.2-14 ng/g) for flounder (*Platichthis flesus*). These levels were comparable to levels measured in fish near the coast of southwest Greenland and in the North Atlantic Ocean. Livers of cod from the coast of southwest Greenland contained 32.4 ng/g on average, and those of hake (*Merluccius merluccius*) from the North Atlantic Ocean averaged 40.5 ng/g) (Ernst, 1986). Levels of HCB were below the determination limit (DL) in cod liver (DL = 5 ng/g) and herring muscle (DL = 1 ng/g) of fish from the Clyde Sea near Scotland (Kelly & Campbell, 1994). Cod from the Firth of Forth had mean liver levels of 38.7 ng/g wet weight, and levels in herring muscle of 2.0 and 2.3 ng/g wet weight were observed in fish from the Firth of Forth and North Sea, respectively (Kelly & Campbell, 1994). In surveillance monitoring of contaminants in fish from coastal waters near England and Wales, concentrations of HCB in livers of cod (*Gadus morhua*), whiting (*Merlangius merlangus*), dab (*Limanda limanda*) and flounder (*Platichthys flesus*) were 2-290, 5-230, 3-55 and 1-52 ng/g, respectively (all results on a wet tissue weight basis) (MAFF/HSE, 1994). Levels of HCB in muscle tissues of herring (*Clupea harengus*) from the Baltic Sea ranged from <1 to 39 ng/g (Hansen et al., 1985); concentrations in whitefish (*Coregonus lavaretus*) and trout (*Salmo trutta*) ranged from <1 to 9 ng/g fresh weight in a 1992 survey (Atuma et al., 1993).

Fish taken from the contaminated waters of the Frierfjord in Norway contained mean concentrations of HCB in liver of 11 600 ng/g for saithe (*Pollachius virens*), and 16 800 ng/g for cod (*Gadus morhua*) (Bjerk & Brevik, 1980). Levels of HCB from fish taken from the uncontaminated Sogndalfjord were much lower, averaging 18 ng/g wet weight in livers of cod (*Gadus morhua*), 8 ng/g in haddock (*Melanogrammus aeglefinus*) and 1 ng/g in lemon sole (*Microstomus kitt*) and flounder (*Platichthys flesus*) (Skåre et al., 1985). Flounder

(*Platichthis flesus*) taken from the Elbe Estuary in Germany, downstream from Hamburg (a highly industrialized area), contained mean levels of HCB in muscle of 688 ng/g (range 84-1907 ng/g wet weight). Further downstream, towards the mouth of the river, levels were lower, averaging 12.5 ng/g (range 2-32 ng/g) (Kohler et al., 1986).

The mean level of HCB in 15 snapping turtle eggs from Ontario, Canada was 27.1 ng/g wet weight (Bishop et al., 1995).

The levels of HCB in birds have been similar across the various regions of Canada since the 1980s, probably as a combined result of emission reductions and the long-range transport of HCB to remote locations. Mean concentrations of HCB in herring gull eggs (*Larus argentatus*) in 1991 ranged from 16 to 71 ng/g wet weight at various colonies in the Great Lakes, and were relatively uniform across lakes (Environment Canada/Department of Fisheries and Oceans/Health and Welfare Canada, 1991). These levels were approximately an order of magnitude lower than in 1974. The mean level of HCB in herring gull eggs from Norwegian coastal waters in 1981 was 120 ng/g wet weight (Moksnes & Norheim, 1986). In a study from the Netherlands, mean levels in eggs of common terns collected in 1987 were 0.03 µg/g wet weight and in those of black-headed gulls collected in 1988 were 93 µg/g fat (Stronkhorst et al., 1993). Levels of HCB found in eggs of sea-bird species (*Haematopus ostralegus, Larus ridibundus, Larus argentatus* and *Sterna hirundo*) from the banks of a river near an organochlorine chemical plant in Germany were ≤ 500 ng/g wet weight (Heidmann, 1986); mean levels of less than 15 ng/g wet weight were found in eggs of several species of land birds, including rooks (*Corvus frugilerus*) and sparrow hawks (*Accipiter nisus*) from agricultural, industrial and rural sites. Recent surveys have indicated similar levels of HCB in the eggs of five other predatory bird species across Canada (means ranged from 10 to 53 ng/g wet weight) (Noble & Elliott, 1986; Pearce et al., 1989; Noble et al., 1992). However, the mean level of HCB in peregrine falcon (*Falco peregrinus*) eggs collected across Canada from 1980 to 1987 was 279 ng/g wet weight, and concentrations ranged as high as 1060 ng/g wet weight (Peakall et al., 1990).

HCB has been found to accumulate in lipids of the common goldeneye duck (*Bucephala clangula*) that overwinter in the Niagara River (mean of 150 ng/g) (Foley & Batcheller, 1988) and the Detroit

River (mean of 1700 ng/g) (Smith et al., 1985a) in the USA. Goldeneye wintering in the Baltic Sea contained average levels of 250 ng/g lipid (Falandysz & Szefer, 1982). Levels of HCB in the livers of silver seagulls taken from estuaries in Germany were lower in 1988 than 1989 (approximately 80 and 150 ng/g fat, respectively, in samples from the River Ems estuary). Higher levels were observed for both years in liver samples of birds taken from the River Elbe estuary (>250 ng/g fat) (BUA 1994).

In breast muscle tissue samples from various species of birds, HCB concentrations tend to be progressively greater at higher trophic levels (i.e., piscivores > molluscivores > omnivores > grazers) (Environment Canada/Department of Fisheries and Oceans/Health and Welfare Canada, 1991).

In the blubber of marine mammals in the Canadian Arctic, mean levels of HCB were 19 ng/g wet weight for ringed seals (*Phoca hispida*) and 491 ng/g wet weight for beluga whales (*Delphinapterus leucas*) (Norstrom et al., 1990), while male belugas sampled in the Gulf of St. Lawrence contained up to 1340 ng/g (Béland et al., 1991). Blubber from male and female white-beaked dolphins (*Lagerorhunchus albirostris*) collected near the Newfoundland coast averaged 1110 ng/g and 880 ng/g wet weight, respectively. Lower levels (290 ng/g and 100 ng/g wet weight) were observed in blubber from male and female pilot whales (*Globicephala meleana*), also collected near the Newfoundland coast (Muir et al., 1988). The higher levels observed in the dolphins may reflect greater exposure to HCB because of overwintering and feeding in the Gulf of St. Lawrence. Blubber of harbour porpoises (*Phocoena phocoena*) collected in Poland between 1989 and 1990 contained an average of 573 ng/g wet weight (Kannan et al., 1993), and those collected around the coast of Scotland between 1989 and 1991 contained an average of 263 ng/g (Wells et al., 1994). Levels of HCB in the blubber of bottlenosed dolphins also collected off the coast of Scotland contained an average of 276 ng/g (Wells et al., 1994). Levels in the blubber of three species of dolphins from the Bay of Bengal, southern India, were low, ranging from 1.1 to 13 ng/g wet weight (Tanabe et al., 1993). Harbour seals (*Phoca vitulina*) found sick or dead in Norwegian waters due to a disease outbreak caused by a morbilli virus had a mean HCB level in the blubber of 27 ng/g wet weight (range of 5-94 ng/g) (Skaare et al., 1990).

Limited data were found on levels of HCB in terrestrial mammals. In a 1973-1974 survey of HCB in the adipose tissue of fox (*Vulpes vulpes*), doe (*Capreolus capreolus*) and wild boar (*Sus scrofa*) in Germany, HCB concentrations ranged from <10 to 3110 ng/g. The lowest levels were observed in the does, presumably because they are herbivorous, whereas foxes and wild boar feed on small animals and are therefore more affected by biomagnification of HCB (Koss & Manz, 1976). Similar patterns were evident in a study from Sweden, in which rabbits (*Oryctolagus cuniculus*, muscle), moose (*Alcaes alcaes,* muscle), reindeer (*Rangifer tarandus,* suet) and osprey (*Pandion haliaetus,* muscle) were found to contain 9, 15, 51 and 330 ng HCB/g lipid weight, respectively (Jansson et al., 1993). The mean concentration in 66 serum samples taken in muskoxen in the Canadian Northwest Territories in 1989 was 2.8 ng/g (range of 1.1-7.5 ng/g) (Salisbury et al., 1992). The mean concentration of HCB in fat samples from 58 caribou from the same region ranged from 32.93 to 129.4 ng/g (lipid corrected) (Elkin & Bethke, 1995). The mean concentration of HCB in the livers and lipids of adult river otters (*Lutra canadensis*) in western Canada were 3 ng/g and 30 ng/g wet weight, respectively, for females and 4 ng/g and 25 ng/g wet weight, respectively, for males (Somers et al., 1987). Concentrations of HCB in mink carcasses collected in Ontario in the late 1970s and early 1980s ranged from < 0.5 to 10 ng/g wet weight (Proulx et al., 1987). In the Canadian north, the mean level of HCB in the fat of polar bears (*Ursus maritimus*) hunted between 1982 and 1984 was 296 ng/g wet weight (Norstrom et al., 1990).

5.1.6 *Food and drinking-water*

HCB is commonly detected, at low levels, in food (Table 7). Levels of HCB tend to be highest in fatty foods and/or those that have been treated with HCB-contaminated pesticides. The most extensive data identified have been collected through the United States Food and Drug Administration (US FDA) Total Diet Study. The results of the surveys from 1982 to 1991 indicate that HCB is detectable (DL = 0.1 ng/g) in a small fraction of food items, most often dairy products, meats, and peanuts/peanut butter (KAN-DO Office and Pesticides Team, 1995). In the most recent surveys, conducted during 1990-1991, mean levels were less than 1 ng/g for all products.

Table 7. Concentration (μg/kg wet weight unless otherwise specified) of hexachlorobenzene in various foods

Country	Food	Mean content[a]	Range	Reference
Australia	cereals	0.01	< 0.01-0.01	Kannan et al. (1994)
	pulses	0.02	0.01-0.05	
	oils	0.07	0.02-0.11	
	beverages	0.03	0.02-0.04	
	vegetables	0.01	< 0.01-0.02	
	fruits	0.01	< 0.01-0.02	
	dairy products	0.55	0.14-1.6	
	meat and fat	0.46	0.01-3.0	
	fishes	4.2	< 0.01-60	
Canada	fresh meat & eggs	0.17		Davies (1988)[b]
	root vegetables & potato	0.04		
	fresh fruit	ND(<0.01)		
	leafy/other above-ground vegetables	0.02		
	2% milk	0.16		
Canada	apples	ND(<0.2)-2.6		OMAF/OME (1988)
	peaches	ND(<0.2)		
	tomatoes	ND(<0.2)		
	potatoes	ND(<0.2)		
	wheat	ND(<0.2)		
	eggs	ND(<0.2)		
	hamburger	0.39	0.2-0.57	
	prime beef		ND(<0.2)-0.21	
	pork	ND(<0.2)		
	chicken	ND(<0.2)		

Table 7 (contd).

Country	Food	Mean content[a]	Range	Reference
Germany	milk	0.22[d]	0.088-0.45[d]	Fürst et al. (1992)
	cream	0.98[d]	0.31-1.30[d]	
	butter	4.86[d]	2.32-6.88[d]	
	cheese	2.72[d]	2.16-3.70[d]	
India	cereals	0.03	0.01-0.04	Kannan et al. (1992a)
	pulses (edible seeds of legumes)	0.07	0.02-0.16	
	spices	0.22	<0.01-0.54	
	oils	1.5	0.09-2.8	
	milk	0.03	0.01-0.10	
	butter	1.7	0.86-2.4	
	fishes & prawn	0.07	<0.01-0.55	
	meat & animal fat	0.61	0.02-4.8	
Mexico	cheese	16.67[d]	1	Albert et al. (1990)
Morocco	eggs	20.9	0.09-300	Kessabi et al. (1990)
	poultry liver	5.1	trace-30.0	
	bovine liver	21.9	1.2-119.8	
	bovine kidney	15.1	trace-133.0	

Table 7 (contd).

Papua New Guinea	cheese	0.43		Kannan et al. (1994)
	pork fat	0.40		
	chicken	0.20		
	striped mullet	0.04	0.02-0.05	
	tilapia	0.01	< 0.01-0.02	
	mud crab	0.03	< 0.01-0.05	
	oyster	0.02		
Solomon Islands	pork	0.14		Kannan et al. (1994)
	chicken	0.06		
	greenspotted kingfish	0.03	0.01-0.06	
	indian mackerel	0.01	0.01	
	paddletail snapper	0.01	0.01	
Southern Baltic	canned cod-livers	60 ± 6	50-76	Falandysz et al. (1993)
Spain	bologna - fresh	2.57[d]		Ariño et al. (1992)
	- cooked	2.48[d]		
Spain	pork sausage			Ariño et al. (1992)
	- before curing	6.63[d]		
	- after 30 days curing	6.0[d]		
Spain	ham - fresh	3.46[d]		Ariño et al. (1992)
	- cured	1.29[d]		
Spain	pork	2.86-3.9[d]		Ariño et al. (1993)

Table 7 (contd).

Country	Food	Mean content[a]	Range	Reference
Spain	lamb - chop, raw	14.67[d]		Conchello et al. (1993)
	- chop, grilled	12.06[d]		
	- leg, raw	8.53[d]		
	- leg, roasted	7.02[d]		
Spain	chicken	120 ± 10		To-Figueras et al. (1986)
	calf	249 ± 37		
	rabbit	860 ± 159		
	pork	169 ± 20		
	sheep	225 ± 35		
	butter	315 ± 18		
United Kingdom	bread	ND (10)		MAFF/HSE (1994)
	milk	0.6		
	butter	ND(10)		
	cheese	3.33[d]		
	ewes' cheese	ND(10)		
	pasta	ND(10)		
	beef burgers	ND(10)		
	canned meat	10[d]		
	cooked meats	10[d]		
	lamb	ND(10)		
	rabbit	ND(10)		
	salami	ND(10)		

Table 7 (contd).

United Kingdom	sausages	ND(10)		MAFF/HSE (1994)
	pies and pasties	ND(10)		
	salmon (tinned)	2.0		
	breaded cod	ND(2.0)		
	fish cakes	2.0		
	mackerel	20		
	plaice	ND(2.0)		
	prawn products	ND(2.0)		
	sardines (tinned)	ND(2.0)		
United Kingdom	carrot	0.0317		Wang & Jones (1994)
	potato	3.35		
	cabbage	0.0418		
	cauliflower	0.0729		
	lettuce	0.108		
	onion	0.0014		
	bean	0.0101		
	pea	0.0039		
	tomato	0.0139		
USA	cheese, processed	0.2	ND-0.5	US FDA (unpublished)[c]
	cheese, cheddar	0.1	ND-0.5	
	beef, ground (regular)	0.1	ND-0.4	
	beef, chuck roast	0.3	ND-1.0	
	beef, round steak	0.2	ND-1.0	
	beef, loin/sirloin steak	0.2	ND-1.0	

Table 7 (contd).

Country	Food	Mean content[a]	Range	Reference
USA	lamb chop	0.3	ND-1.0	US FDA (unpublished)[c]
	frankfurters	0.1	ND-0.6	
	cod/haddock fillet	ND(0.1)	ND-0.2	
	eggs, scrambled	0.1	ND-0.3	
	eggs, fried	0.2	ND-0.7	
	peanut butter	0.2	ND-0.4	
	peanuts, dry roasted	0.3	ND-1.0	
	watermelon	0.1	ND-0.5	
	butter	0.6	ND-1.0	
	cream	0.1	ND-0.4	
Viet Nam	rice	0.03	<0.01-0.05	Kannan et al. (1992b)
	pulses	0.04	<0.01-0.18	
	oil	1.2		
	butter	5.0		
	animal fat	0.41	0.29-0.65	
	meat	0.11	0.03-0.18	
	fish	0.05	0.01-0.31	
	prawn	0.03		
	shellfish	0.04		
	crab	0.17		
	caviar	3.8	1.9-7.2	

[a] ND = not detected (detection limit given in brackets).
[b] Fresh produce and meats grown in Ontario were purchased from four grocery stores in Toronto when locally grown produce was available (Ontario freshwater fish were not available and therefore, were excluded from analysis). All food items were grouped into one of five composites for analysis, with the relative proportions of different food items in each composite calculated from the estimates of the amounts purchased per person per year by Ontario residents.
[c] The US Food and Drug Administration Total Diet Study conducted from April 1990 to April 1991; reporting residue levels in 234 individual food items collected from 3 cities in each of 4 geographical regions of the USA (data available from US FDA, Washington, DC).
[d] Originally reported on a fat basis, and subsequently converted to wet weight using percentage fat contents reported in NHW (1987).

In a number of more limited recent surveys, HCB levels have been determined in commercial foods available in several countries from North America, Europe and Asia (Table 7). The results of these studies are consistent with the USA study described above, in that HCB has been detected primarily in fatty foods such as meats and dairy products. In these studies, mean concentrations are generally in the low ng/g range or less, although substantially higher concentrations have been reported in some surveys from Europe and Asia.

The effects of cooking, curing and ripening on the HCB residues in pork meat products were investigated in Spain by Ariño et al. (1992). Neither cooking at 80-82 °C for 100 min nor curing reduced the HCB content in pork bologna and pork sausage, respectively, whereas the level of HCB in dry-salted and cured ham declined by 42% throughout maturation.

HCB has been detected infrequently, and at very low concentrations in drinking-water supplies (Table 5). Samples of drinking-water collected in 1980 from Canadian cities in the vicinity of Lake Ontario contained from 0.06 to 0.20 ng/litre, with a mean of 0.1 ng/litre (Oliver & Nicol, 1982). In other Canadian and USA surveys, HCB was not detected (US EPA 1985b - DL = 100 ng/litre; Environment Canada, 1989 - DL = 2 ng/litre). Slightly higher concentrations of HCB (median of 1-2 ng/litre) were reported in Croatian drinking-water supplies drawn from a nearby polluted river (pollution sources were not identified) (Fingler et al., 1992).

5.2 General population exposure

5.2.1 Human tissues and fluids

Owing to its persistence and lipophilicity, HCB is present at low levels in the fatty tissues of virtually all members of the general population. Levels of HCB in adipose tissues, breast milk, blood and follicular fluid of various populations from around the world are shown in Table 8. It should be noted that the quality of the studies given in Table 8 varies quite widely, from extensive national surveys to those with relatively few samples.

Levels of HCB in human adipose tissue from around the world are generally <1 mg/kg (Table 8). Although available data are limited, concentrations of HCB reported in fat tissue are generally slightly higher in samples from European countries than from elsewhere in the world. The highest levels reported in recent surveys are from Spain (mean levels of approximately 3-6 mg/kg); the authors suggested that this reflected contamination of foods caused by its presence as an impurity in other pesticides (Camps et al., 1989; Gómez-Catalán et al., 1993, 1995). Concentrations of HCB increased with age in a number of these surveys, but there were no consistent differences in residue levels between the sexes (Mes et al., 1982; Williams et al., 1984, 1988; Abbott et al., 1985; Mes, 1990; Mes et al., 1990; Gomez-Catalan et al., 1993; Kemper, 1993; Ludwicki & Góralczyk, 1994).

In general, concentrations of HCB in breast milk in various countries or regions (Table 8) range widely, and appear to be related to the degree of industrialization and/or urbanization within the survey area. The levels of HCB in breast milk have been expressed on a whole milk basis, using the fat content reported by the authors or, where this was not reported, a fat content of 4.2% (NHW, 1987). Schechter et al. (1989a) reported that concentrations of HCB in breast milk in the mid-1980s were lowest in samples from Thailand (0.3 µg/litre whole milk) and Viet Nam (< 0.17 µg/litre), somewhat higher in those from a semi-rural area of the USA (0.7-0.8 µg/litre), and higher still in German samples (12.6 µg/litre) (numbers of samples in this study were extremely small, except for the German data (n=167)). In surveys summarized by Mes et al. (1986), mean HCB levels were 1 µg/litre whole milk in the USA, 2 µg/litre in Canada, 3 µg/litre in Sweden, 4 µg/litre in Great Britain, and 35µg/litre in Germany. Still higher levels (48-89 µg/litre whole milk) have been reported in studies from Spain (Conde et al. 1993). Bates et al. (1994) reported that the concentrations of HCB in breast milk of primiparae from New Zealand increased linearly with age, but were not related to body mass index, fish intake, smoking status, type of residential water supply or location of residence (urban versus rural). In a study of body burdens of organochlorines in an indigenous population, Ayotte et al. (1995) reported that mean concentrations of HCB in the milk fat of 107 Inuit women from northern Quebec were several times higher than those in 50 Caucasian women from southern Quebec (57 and 1.2 µg/litre whole milk, respectively). Levels of organochlorine compounds in breast milk correlated with levels of omega-3 fatty acids in plasma phospholipids, indicating that consumption of marine organisms is an important source of exposure to these xenobiotics.

Table 8. Levels of hexachlorobenzene in human tissues and fluids
(mg/kg wet weight adipose tissue; mg/kg whole milk; µg/litre blood serum; µg/litre follicular fluid)

Country	Sample size	Mean tissue concentration (range)	Year	Reference
A. Adipose tissue				
Australia	31	0.14[a] (0.01-1.70) (fat basis)	1990-1991	Stevens et al. (1993)
Canada	108	0.026[a] (0.0073-0.118)	1985	Mes & Malcolm (1992), Mes et al. (1990)
Canada	25	0.019[a] (max. value: 0.087)	-	Mes (1992)
Canada	141	0.071 (males) (0.018-0.244) 0.109 (females) (0.019-0.373)	1984	Williams et al. (1988)
Canada	99	0.095 (0.01-0.667)	1976	Mes et al. (1982)
Canada	168	0.062 (0.001-0.52)	1972	Mes et al. (1977)
Federal Republic of Germany	93	(0.11-21.8)	1971	Leoni & D'Arca (1976)
Federal Republic of Germany	6	0.263 (0.083-0.753)		van der Ven et al. (1992)
India	7	0.012 (0-0.064)	1987	Nair & Pillai (1989)

Table 8 (contd).

Country	Sample size	Mean tissue concentration (range)	Year	Reference
A. Adipose tissue (contd)				
Italy	28	0.491 (0.126-1.36)	1973-1974	Leoni & D'Arca (1976)
Japan	39	0.044	1986-1987	Kashimoto et al. (1989)
Japan	15	0.21 (0.10-0.42)	-	Morita et al. (1975)
Netherlands	average of 51/year	0.7[a] (fat basis)	1968-1969	Greve & Van Zoonen (1990)
		1.2[a] (fat basis)	1973-1975	
		0.86[a] (fat basis)	1976	
		0.98[a] (fat basis)	1977-1978	
		0.85[a] (fat basis)	1980	
		0.80[a] (fat basis)	1981	
		0.58[a] (fat basis)	1982	
		0.49[a] (fat basis)	1983	
		0.42[a] (fat basis)	1985	
		0.38[a] (fat basis)	1986	
New Zealand	-	0.31	-	US EPA (1985a)
Poland	53	0.221 (0.068-0.937)	early 1980s	Szymczyński et al. (1986)
Poland	277	0.31	1989-1992	Ludwicki & Góralczyk (1994)

Table 8 (contd).

A. Adipose tissue (contd)				
Spain (4 cities)	256	2.99	1985-1988	Gómez-Catalán et al. (1993)
Spain	86	3.37 (0.42-12.53) (lipid basis)	1991	Gómez-Catalán et al. (1995)
Spain	171	5.55	1982-1983	To-Figueras et al. (1986)
Spain	168	2.95 (0.2-17.37)	1988-89	Ferrer et al. (1992)
United Republic of Tanzania	9	0.003 (0.0013-0.0076)	-	van der Ven et al. (1992
United Kingdom	201	0.05 (n.d-0.29)	1969-1971	Abbott et al. (1972)
United Kingdom	236	0.19 (0.02-3.2)	1976-1977	Abbott et al. (1981)
United Kingdom	187	0.11 (0.03-0.32)	1982-1983	Abbott et al. (1985)
USA	10	0.125 (0.03-0.47	-	Barquet et al. (1981)
USA	6081	0.037[a]	1974-1983	Robinson et al. (1990)

Table 8 (contd).

Country	Sample size	Mean tissue concentration (range)	Year	Reference
A. Adipose tissue (contd)				
USA	763 689 671	0.118 (0.001-0.256) 0.043 (0.032-0.054) 0.051 (0.043-0.059)	1982 1984 1986	US EPA (1994)
B. Breast milk[b]				
Australia	39 28	0.042 (rural) 0.063 (urban)	1970	Newton & Greene (1972)
Australia	137 130	0.007 (0.002-0.019) (rural) 0.008 (0.002-0.017) (urban)	1979-1980	Stacey et al. (1985)
Australia	60	0.017 (0.0007-0.32)	-	Quinsey et al. (1995)
Australia	128	0.0036[a] (<0.01-0.216)	1990-1991	Stevens et al. (1993)
Brazil	30	0.00048 (0.00024-0.0036)[c]	1987-1988	Beretta & Dick (1994)
Canada	412	0.0008 (max = 0.014)	1986	Mes et al. (1993)
Canada	210	0.002 (max.= 0.009)	1982	Mes et al. (1986)
Canada	100	0.002 (max.= 0.021)	1975	Mes & Davies (1979)

Table 8 (contd).

B. Breast milk[b] (contd)				
Canada	536	0.0013[c]	1989-1990	Dewailly et al. (1991)
Canada	127	0.00051	1978	Frank et al. (1988)
	15	0.0004	1979	
	12	0.00028	1980-1981	
	13	0.00052	1983-1984	
	18	0.00026	1985	
Finland	143[c]	0.002[c]	1984-1985	Mussalo-Rauhamaa et al. (1988)
Finland	50	0.0023 (0.0007-0.006)	1982	Wickström et al. (1983)
France	20	0.002 (0.00004-0.008)[c]	1990-1991	Bordet et al. (1993)
Federal Republic of Germany	144	0.021[c]	1984	Fürst et al. (1994)
	220	0.019[c]	1985	
	157	0.015[c]	1986	
	144	0.015[c]	1987	
	196	0.013[c]	1988	
	145	0.01[c]	1989	
	286	0.0095[c]	1990	
	113	0.0074[c]	1991	
Federal Republic of Germany	167	0.0126[c]	1985-1987	Schecter et al. (1989a)

Table 8 (contd).

Country	Sample size	Mean tissue concentration (range)	Year	Reference
B. Breast milk[b] (contd)				
Federal Republic of Germany	2709	0.048[c]	1979-1981	BUA (1994)
	3778	0.013[c]	1986	
	1897	0.014[c]	1987	
	2994	0.011[c]	1988	
	3256	0.01[c]	1989	
	5340	0.009[c]	1990	
Former German Democratic Republic	483	0.007[c]	1990-1991	
India	16	0.042 (0-0.25)[e]	1987	Nair & Pillai (1989)
Israel	100	0.00256	-	Weisenberg et al. (1985)
Italy	56	0.058[d]	-	Franchi & Focardi (1991)
Italy	64	0.006 (0.004-0.009)	1987	Larsen et al. (1994)
Netherlands	202	0.036[a,c]	1972-1973	Greve & Van Zoonen (1990)
	278	0.008[a,c]	1983	
New Zealand	38	0.0011	1988	Bates et al. (1994)

Table 8 (contd).

B. Breast milk[b] (contd)				
Norway	28	0.0007	1991	Johansen et al. (1994)
Spain	240 358	0.089(0.039-0.21)[c] 0.048(0.037-0.073)[c]	1984-1987 1990-1991	Conde et al. (1993)
Sweden	20	0.0042 (0.002-0.009)[c]	1978	Norén (1983a)
Sweden	2	0.0007-0.004[c]	-	Norén (1983b)
Sweden	227 245 340 102	0.003 (0.002-0.004)[c] 0.003 (0.003-0.004)[c] 0.003 (0.003-0.004)[c] 0.001 (0.0008-0.001)[c]	1972 1976 1980 1984-1985	Norén (1988)
Sweden	140	0.0012[c]	1989	Norén (1993)
Sweden	40	0.0017[c]	1986-1987	Vaz et al. (1993)
Thailand	3	0.0003[c]	1985-1987	Schecter et al. (1989a)
Turkey	51	0.0035[c]	1988	Üstünbas et al. (1994)
Turkey	56	0.021[c]	20-30 years post-exposure during 1955-1959	Gocmen et al. (1989)

Table 8 (contd).

Country	Sample size	Mean tissue concentration (range)	Year	Reference
B. Breast milk[b] (contd)				
United Kingdom	193	0.001 (<0.001-0.005)	1989-1991	MAFF (1992)
USA	40	0.00052	1979	Bush et al. (1985)
USA	8	0.0007-0.0008[c]	1985-1987	Schecter et al. (1989a)
Viet Nam	12	<0.00017[c]	1985-1987	Schecter et al. (1989a)
Yugoslavia	10	0.006 (0.002-0.017)	1978	Kodric-Smit et al. (1980)
C. Serum				
Canada	25 29 20	0.25 0.21 0.35	1993	Jarrel et al. (1993)
Croatia	15 24 26 32	1[a] (<0.5-4) 0.9[a] (<0.5-3) 1[a] (<0.5-7) <0.5[a] (<0.5-4)	1985 1987-1988 1989-1990 1990	Krauthacker (1993)
Germany	6	1.23 (0.33-2.66)[f]	-	van der Ven et al. (1992)

Table 8 (contd).

C. Serum (contd)				
Spain (near organochlorine compounds factory)	21	26 (7.5-69)	1992	Grimalt et al. (1994)
Spain (hospital in Barcelona)	13	4.8 (1.5-15)	1992	Grimalt et al. (1994)
Spain	100	11.09 (1.60-94.2) 4.13 (0.70-19.7)	1986 1993-1994	To-Figueras et al. (1995)
United Republic of Tanzania	11	0.01 (0-0.03)[f]	-	van der Ven et al. (1992)
USA	370	0.189[a] (0.05-3.21)	-	Needham et al. (1990)
D. Whole blood				
Slovakia	50	25.2 (6.1-43.2)	1992	Kočan et al. (1994)

Table 8 (contd).

Country	Sample size	Mean tissue concentration (range)	Year	Reference
E. Follicular fluid				
Canada	25 29 20	0.11 0.14 0.20	1993	Jarrell et al. (1993b)
Federal Republic of Germany	15	2.59 (1.1-5.7)	-	Trapp et al. (1984)

[a] Median value.
[b] The most recent data were used for calculation of intakes via breast milk (section 5.2.4).
[c] Originally expressed as mg/kg milk fat and subsequently converted to a wet weight basis using either the % fat reported, or if not given, using 4.2% fat (NHW, 1987).
[d] Number of positive samples
[e] Originally expressed on a dry weight basis and subsequently converted to wet weight using 88% moisture for conversion (NHW, 1987).
[f] Values reported in µg/kg.

In a HCB poisoning incident in Turkey (section 8.1), breast-fed infants were fatally intoxicated through their mothers' milk. In an early report of this incident (Peters et al., 1966), HCB was reported as being present in breast milk, although it was not quantified. However, elevated levels were measured (mean of 510 ng/g on a fat basis (approximately 21 ng/g on a wet weight basis) for 56 porphyric mothers) 20-30 years after the incident, compared with a mean of 70 ng/g fat in 77 milk samples from women of families without porphyria or from areas outside of the endemic area (Peters et al., 1982; Gocmen et al., 1989).

HCB is present in a wide range of other tissues and fluids from humans, but at lower levels than in adipose tissue and breast milk. For example, concentrations of HCB in serum of 370 subjects from the general population in the USA studied by Needham et al. (1990) averaged 0.189 μg/litre, compared to concentrations of 39 ng/g lipid in 287 adipose tissue samples. Schechter et al. (1989b) reported HCB levels in various organs in autopsy tissue from three American patients. HCB levels in adipose tissue ranged from 15 to 24 ng/g wet tissue, while kidney, muscle, lung, spleen and testis contained 1 ng/g or less, and adrenals, bone marrow and liver contained intermediate concentrations.

Median blood serum levels of HCB ranged from <0.5 to 1.0 μg/litre in four population groups (total of 97 samples) from Zagreb, Croatia (Krauthacker, 1993). The groups included workers employed in the distribution and packing of seeds treated with different pesticides, who were expected to have absorbed organochlorine compounds at levels greater than the general population. However, levels of HCB in the blood of these workers were not elevated. Van der Ven et al. (1992) reported the HCB levels in maternal serum of 6 and 11 full-term pregnant women in Germany and Tanzania, respectively. Levels in Germany averaged 1.23 μg/kg (0.33-2.66 μg/kg), whereas those in Tanzania were 0.01 μg/kg (0-0.03 μg/kg). Analysis of blood plasma samples from a human organ specimen bank in Germany revealed that median annual concentrations of HCB between 1983 and 1989 ranged between 3.1 and 5.4 μg/litre (Kemper, 1993). Serum and ovarian follicular fluid have been shown to contain HCB in patients receiving *in vitro* fertilization (Jarrell et al., 1993b). Of 72 patients, HCB was detected in the serum of 60 and follicular fluid of 49. There was a significant geographical variation among three major cities in Canada (Jarrell et al., 1993b). Follicular fluid from similarly treated patients in Germany has been shown to contain HCB (Trapp et al., 1994). In some studies, workers exposed to chlorinated solvents or chlorinated pesticides had elevated levels of HCB in blood (section 5.2.7).

5.2.2 Intake from ambient air

Based on a daily inhalation volume for adults of 22 m^3, a mean body weight for males and females of 64 kg (IPCS, 1994), and the range of mean levels of HCB measured in ambient air in cities from around the world of approximately 0.1 to 0.6 ng/m^3 (Table 4), mean intake of HCB from ambient air for the general population is estimated to range from 3.4×10^{-5} to 2.1×10^{-4} μg/kg body weight per day. Since no data on levels of HCB in indoor air were found, it has been assumed that levels indoors are the same as those outdoors. The intake of HCB via air may be greater in populations residing in the vicinity of point sources, but this exposure is considered to be too site-specific to estimate reliably.

5.2.3 Intake from drinking-water

Based on a daily volume of ingestion for adults of 1.4 litres, a mean body weight for males and females of 64 kg (IPCS, 1994), and the range of mean concentrations of HCB detected in drinking-water from cities of approximately 0.1 to 2 ng/litre (Table 5), the estimated mean daily intake of HCB from drinking water for the general population ranges from approximately 2.2×10^{-6} to 4.4×10^{-5} μg/kg body weight per day.

5.2.4 Intake from foods

Based on the average daily consumption of various foodstuffs by adults from around the world[a], a mean body weight for males and females of 64 kg (IPCS, 1994), and the mean level of HCB detected

[a] Dietary intakes (g/person/day) consist of: cereals, 323, starchy roots, 225; sugar (excludes syrups and honey), 72; pulses and nuts, 33; vegetables and fruits, 325; meat, 125; eggs, 19; fish, 23; milk products (excludes butter), 360; fats and oils (includes butter), 31 (all intakes from IPCS, 1994).

in various foods in the 1990-1991 US FDA Total Diet Study (Table 7), the estimated daily intake of HCB from food ranges from approximately 0.0004 to 0.0028 µg/kg body weight per day (this range was generated by assuming, for food groups in which HCB was not detected, that non-detectable values were zero with the detection limit being 0.1 µg/kg. These estimates overlap the range of dietary estimates (between 0.001 and 0.027 µg/kg body weight per day) that have been reported for various countries (Canada, USA., Germany, Finland, Viet Nam, Thailand, India, Japan, Australia, the Netherlands) (Gartrell et al., 1986; De Walle et al., 1995; Fujita & Morikawa, 1992; Kannan et al., 1992a,b; Government of Canada, 1993; Kannan et al., 1994). Intakes via food may be substantially higher in selected European and Asian countries, where the content of HCB in a sampling of a limited range of foods was relatively high (Table 7), or in indigenous populations consuming large quantities of some wildlife species, such as marine mammals, that are known to accumulate relatively high tissue levels of lipophilic contaminants (Government of Canada, 1993; Ayotte et al., 1995; Kuhnlein et al., 1995).

Dietary intakes may also be greater in infants during breast-feeding, owing to the accumulation of HCB in the mothers' milk. The mean concentrations of HCB in the most recent surveys found for various countries range from <0.17 to 48 µg HCB/litre whole milk (Table 8). Assuming that infants are exclusively breast fed for the first 6 months, during which they consume an average of 0.75 litres of breast milk per day and have an average body weight of 7 kg (Health Canada, 1994), the estimated mean intakes of HCB from breast milk in various countries range from <0.018 to 5.1 µg/kg body weight per day. Daily intakes of HCB by breast-feeding infants of Inuit mothers in northern Quebec, Canada (a population that consumes substantial quantities of marine organisms that accumulate lipophilic contaminants) was estimated at 0.45 µg/kg body weight per day, a value that was several times greater than for a more southerly population in the same province (Ayotte et al., 1995).

5.2.5 *Apportionment of intakes*

Total intake of HCB from ambient air, drinking-water and foods is estimated to range from approximately 0.0004 to 0.003 µg/kg body weight per day for the general population, the principal route of exposure being through the diet (92%). The estimated contributions from air and drinking-water are much smaller (7% and 1%, respectively). (The contribution from each environmental medium was calculated based on the mid-point of the intakes estimated in the previous sections.)

5.2.6 Trends in exposure of the general population over time

The results of most studies of the levels of HCB in foods and human tissues over time indicate that exposure of the general population to HCB declined from the 1970s to the mid-1990s in many locations. However, this trend has not been evident during the last decade in some other locations.

Routine monitoring of foods in some countries indicates that exposure to HCB is decreasing. For example, mean concentrations in grab samples of milk, bovine fat, poultry fat and egg fat collected from suppliers in Ontario, Canada, decreased by an order of magnitude or more between the early 1970s and the mid-1980s (Frank et al., 1983, 1985a, 1985b; Frank & Ripley, 1990). Brown et al. (1986) reported that the frequency of detectable (> 10 ng/g in fat samples, wet weight) levels of HCB in the USA meat and poultry supply increased dramatically from 1972 to 1977-1978, but had fallen off sharply up to 1984. More recent data collected through the US FDA Total Diet Study indicate that this trend had continued. Between 1982-1984 and 1991, the most recent year for which data are available, both the frequency of detection of HCB and the estimated average daily intake for people of various ages decreased by roughly 80% (US FDA 1990, 1991, 1992). A decline in HCB levels in fish from the Baltic and the Swedish West Coast was found in the National Swedish Monitoring Programme over the period 1988 to 1994 (Bignert, 1995). The annual decrease in levels in herring muscle from different places in the Baltic was 12 to 15% and in cod liver from the Baltic 21%; from the West Coast it was 12% in herring muscle, 23% in cod liver and 23% in dab liver. The trend with higher concentrations in samples from the Baltic as compared to the West Coast is still seen in the samples.

The results of most studies of temporal trends of HCB levels in human adipose tissue or milk (summarized in Table 8) indicate that general population exposures have declined since the 1970s. In routine monitoring of breast milk contaminants in German mothers, mean concentrations of HCB declined by more than 50% between 1984 and 1991 (Fürst et al., 1994), and by about 80% between 1979 and 1990 (BUA 1994). The median HCB content in samples of plasma from a human specimen bank in Germany decreased from 4.8 µg/litre in 1983 to 3.1 µg/litre in 1989, a period of increasing restrictions on indoor applications of pentachlorophenol, which contains HCB as a contaminant (Kemper, 1993). Mes (1990) reported that concentrations of HCB in human adipose tissue from Canadian surveys were significantly lower in 1985 than in 1972; this decrease occurred in all age classes over this period. An increase in the HCB content of human adipose tissue and milk was observed in the early 1970s in the Netherlands, and was attributed to an increase in the HCB concentration in products of animal origin (Greve & Van Zoonen, 1990). Once measures were taken to avoid contamination of such products, a gradual decrease in HCB levels was observed. Johansen et al. (1994) reported that the concentration of HCB in routine monitoring of milk from Norwegian mothers declined by 65% between 1982 and 1991. In contrast, in the most extensive study of levels of HCB in adipose tissues, the US National Human Adipose Tissue Survey (Robinson et al., 1990), in which data on residues were collected from a nationally representative sample of 6081 autopsies and surgical patients from 1974-1983, there was little change in residue concentrations over the study period, with the national median level remaining near 30 to 40 ng/g.

5.2.7 Occupational exposure during manufacture, formulation, or use

Workers may be exposed to higher concentrations of HCB than the general population, particularly in the manufacture of chlorinated solvents, and in the manufacture and application of pesticides contaminated with HCB.

In a survey of production industries (perchloroethylene, trichloroethylene, carbon tetrachloride, chlorine, triazine herbicides and pentachloronitrobenzene), the highest HCB concentrations were associated with the production of perchloroethylene and trichloroethylene (Spigarelli et al., 1986). The highest level of HCB determined in the air on plant property was 24 µg/m^3 at a plant producing perchloroethylene, carbon tetrachloride and chlorine. Relatively high HCB levels (maximum concentration of 2.2 µg/m^3 in air) were also detected in samples from the pentachloronitrobenzene production plant. Lower levels of HCB were measured at triazine herbicide production plants (ND - 0.02 µg/m^3), and, in the one plant that produced only carbon tetrachloride, HCB was not detected (MDL not reported). It is not known how representative the data from these studies are, as the generation and release of HCB would be minimized in plants using appropriate modern technology and waste management practices.

Personal breathing-zone samples (54 in all) from workers in a pentachlorophenol production plant contained HCB concentrations ranging from <0.1 to 120 μg/m^3 (Marlow, 1986), while levels in 112 area samples throughout the plant ranged from <0.1 to 630 μg/m^3.

HCB concentrations in the blood of workers in a factory producing chlorinated solvents ranged from 14 to 233 μg/litre (Burns & Miller, 1975); this compared with a range <1 to 310 μg/litre in the blood of vegetable spraymen (Burns et al., 1974). Mean levels of HCB in the blood plasma of workers in a chlorinated solvents plant in the USA were 311 μg/litre in 1974, and 312 μg/litre in 1975, and levels in whole blood were 160 μg/litre in 1976, and 170 μg/litre in 1977 (Currier et al., 1980). Concentrations of HCB in blood were positively correlated with the number of years worked in the plant, but were not associated with airborne levels of HCB or job-category-based exposure estimates. Pesticide-exposed vineyard workers in Germany tended to have higher HCB whole blood levels (median 7 μg/litre, maximum 30 μg/litre) than reference controls (median 3 μg/litre, maximum 17 μg/litre) (Kemper, 1993). Angerer et al. (1992) reported that the mean plasma level of HCB in 53 workers at a municipal waste incinerator was 5.0 μg/litre, compared with 4.69 μg/litre in 64 subjects with no known occupational contact.

6. KINETICS AND METABOLISM

6.1 Aquatic and terrestrial biota

Terrestrial plants such as barley, cress and wheat, and algae such as *Oedogonium cardiacum* slowly metabolize HCB to polar metabolites and non-extractable residues (Lu & Metcalf, 1975; Scheunert et al., 1983, 1985; Topp et al., 1989). For example, of the total radiolabelled HCB in barley after uptake from soil over one growing season, 14% was present as polar metabolites, 20% as plant-bound residues and the remainder as the parent compound (Topp et al., 1989). In the only available study on HCB depuration rates in plants, the aquatic macrophyte *Myriophyllum spicatum* eliminated 95% of HCB during the first 28 days after exposure ceased (Gobas et al., 1991).

Invertebrates slowly metabolize HCB to compounds such as pentachlorothioanisole, pentachlorophenol and other polar metabolites (Lu & Metcalf, 1975; Bauer et al., 1989). In an aquatic model ecosystem treated with ^{14}C-HCB for 24 h, unchanged HCB accounted for 84% of the total radioactivity in snails (*Physa sp.*), 67% in water fleas (*Daphnia magna*) and 65% in mosquito larvae (*Culex pipiens*) (Lu & Metcalf, 1975). Half-lives for the elimination of HCB by invertebrates were less than 5 days for filter-feeding bivalves (*Elliptio complanata* and *Mytilus edulis*) (Bro-Rasmussen, 1986; Russell & Gobas, 1989), 16 days for deposit-feeding clams (*Macoma nasuta*) (Boese et al., 1990), and 27 days for oligochaete worms (*Tubifex tubifex* and *Limnodrilus hoffmeisteri*) (Oliver, 1987).

Sanborn et al. (1977) detected pentachlorophenol and at least four unidentified polar metabolites in green sunfish (*Lepomis cyanellus*) after 28 days of ingesting HCB-contaminated food. Pentachlorophenol has also been detected in the excreta and tissues of rainbow trout (*Oncorhynchus mykiss*) following an intraperitoneal dose with HCB (Koss & Koransky, 1978; Koss et al., 1978). Zebra fish (*Brachydanio rerio*) did not metabolize HCB after a 48-h exposure in water (Kasokat et al., 1989). Elimination half-lives of HCB ranged from 7-21 days for fathead minnows (*Pimephales promelas*) after a waterborne exposure (Kosian et al., 1981) to up to 210 days for rainbow trout (*Oncorhynchus mykiss*) after ingestion of HCB in food (Niimi & Cho, 1981).

Clark et al. (1987) reported that 63% of the total HCB eliminated in herring gulls (*Larus argentatus*) was found in the egg yolk. Breslin et al. (1983) found that 50% of total HCB eliminated from laying bobwhite quail (*Colinus virginianus*), a species that lays many eggs, was accounted for in egg yolk. For most wild species, egg laying will account for a relatively small loss of HCB, while depletion of stored fat during energetically costly activities such as migration and moulting may result in a significant reduction in body burdens. The half-life for elimination of HCB in birds ranged from 24-35 days for domesticated chickens (*Gallus gallus domesticus*) fed HCB-contaminated diets (Kan & Tuinstra, 1976; Hansen et al., 1978) to 211 days in intraperitoneally dosed juvenile herring gulls (Clark et al., 1987).

6.2 Mammals

There are few data on the absorption of HCB by humans. By comparing intake and faecal excretion of HCB in a single breast-fed infant, Abraham et al (1994) estimated that absorption was virtually complete (greater than 99.7% at one month of age and greater than 97% at 5 months). The concentrations of HCB in the diet and faeces of a single formula-fed infant were too low for reliable estimation of absorption (Abraham et al., 1994). The results of animal studies indicate that 80% or more of an oral dose of HCB (between 10 and 180 mg/kg body weight) is absorbed if administered in an oil vehicle (Albro & Thomas, 1974; Koss & Koransky, 1975; Ingebritsen et al., 1981; Bleavins et al., 1982). In female rats treated with ^{14}C-HCB in oil, peak values of radioactivity were reached in 2 to 5 days. The absorption was poor (2-20%, depending on the dose) when the substance was given as an aqueous suspension (Koss & Koransky, 1975). Little information was identified on dermal absorption, although it appears to be lower. Koizumi (1991) observed that after dermal application of approximately 2.5 mg ^{14}C-HCB in tetrachloroethylene to Fisher-344 rats for 72 h, only 9.7% of the administered dose was absorbed. No information on absorption via the lungs has been reported.

There are no experimental studies of tissue distribution of HCB in humans, although in a small autopsy study of members of the general population (Schechter et al., 1989b), the highest levels were found in (in order) adipose tissue, adrenals, bone marrow and liver.

Laboratory studies in a number of animal species also indicate that the highest concentrations of HCB are accumulated in tissues with a high lipid content, such as the adipose tissue, adrenal cortex, bone marrow, skin and some endocrine tissues (thyroid, adrenal and ovary) following ingestion or injection of HCB (Koss & Koransky, 1975; Yang et al., 1978; Courtney, 1979; Sundlof et al., 1982; Ingebritsen, 1986; Smith et al., 1987, 1994; Goldey et al., 1990; Foster et al., 1993; Jarrell et al., 1993a). No information was found on the tissue distribution following inhalation or dermal exposure. HCB crosses the placenta, and is eliminated via the mothers' milk in both animals and humans (Villeneuve et al., 1974; Mendoza et al., 1975; Courtney & Andrews, 1979, 1985; Courtney et al., 1979; Bailey et al., 1980; Bleavins et al., 1982; Goldey et al., 1990; section 5.2.1).

Metabolic transformation is not extensive in the wide range of species examined. The pathways of biotransformation of HCB have been reviewed by Debets & Strik (1979) and by Renner (1988). The metabolism of HCB operates via three distinct pathways. These are oxidative pathways, which give rise to phenolic metabolites including pentachlorophenol, tetrachlorohydroquinone and tetrachlorobenzoquinone; a glutathione-conjugation pathway leading to pentachlorothiophenol, pentachlorothioanisoles, and several other sulfur-containing metabolites; and a minor pathway that yields lower chlorinated benzenes through reductive dechlorination. Metabolism occurs primarily in the liver, although dechlorination of HCB has also been demonstrated *in vitro* in enzyme preparations from the lung, kidney and small intestine (Mehendale et al., 1975).

The metabolism of HCB has been studied in the rat and guinea-pig (Mehendale et al., 1975; Rozman et al., 1975; Koss & Koransky, 1976; Koss et al., 1978; Koss & Koransky, 1978; Courtney, 1979), and in the monkey (Rozman et al., 1975; Courtney, 1979). Dosing routes included gastric intubation and the intraperitoneal route, while dosing vehicles included oil and aqueous media. The monitoring for metabolic products of HCB has included excretory products and/or tissue residues for periods ranging from 28 to 40 days post-dosing. Findings were quite dissimilar among the studies. The most common finding was that less than 40% of the administered dose was recovered in the excretory products and a majority of the recovered dose was unchanged HCB.

The major metabolites found in the urine of rats, mice and guinea-pigs exposed to HCB by various routes in most studies are pentachlorophenol (PCP), tetrachlorohydroquinone and pentachlorothiophenol (PCTP) (Koss & Koransky, 1978; Koss et al., 1978). (There is some question as to whether most of the latter compound detected in some studies was an analytical artefact from alkaline hydrolysis of the *n*-acetyl cysteine conjugate.) Other metabolites include tetra- and pentachlorobenzenes and thioanisoles, and tri- and tetrachlorophenols, both in free and conjugated forms. It has been reported that, after dietary exposure of male and female Wistar rats to HCB for 13 weeks, *N*-acetyl-*S*-(pentachlorophenyl)cysteine was the most abundant metabolite via the conjugation pathway (89-92% of the total urinary metabolites collected over 24 h, after one week of treatment). Mercaptotetrachlorothioanisole was also present, excreted as a glucuronide (den Besten et al., 1994). The excreta from male Wistar rats given 125 mg/kg body weight on day 1 and 6 were collected for 12 days (Jansson & Bergman, 1978). Faeces and/or urine contained HCB (about 4% of the total does), pentachlorobenzene, pentachlorophenol, pentachlorobenzenethiol (both as such and as conjugates), methylthiopentachlorobenzene, tetrachlorobenzenedithiol and/or methylthiotetrachlorobenzenethiol (both as such and as conjugates), dichlorotetrakis(methylthio)benzene (trace amounts), hexakis(methylthio)benzene (trace amounts), bis(methylthio)tetrachlorobenzene, tetrachlorobenzenethiol (trace amounts) and methylthiotetrachlorobenzene (trace amounts). Compounds found accumulated in adipose tissue were hexachlorobenzene, pentachlorobenzene, pentachlorobenzenethiol, bis(methylthio)tetrachlorobenzene and pentachloroanisole.

Rizzardini & Smith (1982) administered 50 µmoles of HCB/kg body weight to male and female rats by gavage in arachis oil for 103 days. Three urinary metabolites were identified, i.e., pentachlorophenol, 2,3,5,6-tetrachlorobenzene, 1,4-diol and pentachlorothiophenol (derived from mercapturate). The authors reported that female rats excreted several times more HCB metabolites than males.

PCP and PCTP have been detected in the urine of humans from the general population of Spain with high body burdens of HCB (To-Figueras et al., 1992).

No reliable information on the elimination half-life of HCB in humans was found. Excretion of HCB by laboratory animals occurs mainly through the faeces regardless of the route of administration (US EPA, 1985a; ATSDR, 1990). Both biliary excretion and non-biliary intestinal transfer contribute to faecal excretion (Rozman et al., 1981; Ingebritsen et al., 1981; Richter & Schäfer, 1981; Sundlof et al., 1982). Reported half-lives for the elimination of an oral dose of HCB (doses were 3 mg/kg body weight or less in these studies) are approximately one month in rats and rabbits, 10-18 weeks in sheep, pigs and dogs, and 2.5 to 3 years in rhesus monkeys (Avrahami & Steele, 1972; Avrahami, 1975; Rozman et al., 1981; Sundlof et al., 1982; Scheufler & Rozman, 1984; Yamaguchi et al., 1986). HCB has been detected in the milk of several species, including humans, and the results of experiments with mice and ferrets indicate that the majority of the maternal body burden can be eliminated via the mother's milk during lactation (Bleavins et al., 1982; Courtney & Andrews, 1985).

7. EFFECTS ON LABORATORY MAMMALS AND *IN VITRO* TEST SYSTEMS

This section summarizes the extensive literature on the toxicity of HCB to laboratory mammals, with emphasis on those studies reporting the lowest-observed-effect levels. Information on the dosage with respect to body weight was obtained from the original papers, wherever possible. When doses were not expressed in this way by the investigators and could not be calculated from the data provided, approximate doses (given in parentheses) have been estimated based on the reference values given in NIOSH (1985).

7.1 Single exposure

The acute toxicity of HCB in experimental animals is low; reported oral LD_{50} values for various species range from 1700 mg/kg body weight for the cat to between 3500 and > 10 000 mg/kg body weight for the rat, with intermediate values for the mouse, rabbit and guinea-pig. Reported LC_{50} values for inhalation exposure range from 1600 mg/m^3 for the cat to 4000 mg/m^3 for the mouse, with intermediate values reported for the rat and rabbit (IARC, 1979; Strik, 1986; Lewis, 1992). Acute lethal doses elicit convulsions, tremors, weakness, ataxia, paralysis and pathological changes in organs. Strik (1986) reported that HCB has a low skin irritation score, is not irritating to the eye and does not sensitize the guinea-pig, although no details were provided. In several studies, single oral doses of 100-1000 mg/kg body weight produced increases in the activities of various liver enzymes in rats within 24 h (Strik, 1986).

7.2 Short-term and subchronic exposure

The effects of short-term, repeated exposure to HCB are primarily hepatotoxic and neurological. In a number of studies, the effects of HCB on rats exposed to oral doses in the range of 30-250 mg/kg body weight per day included altered body weight, cutaneous lesions, tremors and other neurological signs, hepatomegaly, liver damage and, in some cases, early alterations in porphyrin or haem metabolism (Courtney, 1979; US EPA, 1985a; Strik, 1986). Short-term exposure *in vivo* induced a variety of enzymes, including glutathione-*S*-transferases and isozymes of cytochrome P-450, identified as cytochromes P-450IA1 (CYPIA1), P-450IA2 (CYPIA2) and P-450IIB

(CYPIIB) (Wada et al., 1968; Courtney, 1979; Denomme et al., 1983; US EPA, 1985a; Linko et al., 1986; Strik, 1986; Hahn et al., 1988, 1989; Vos et al., 1988; Green et al., 1989; Rizzardini et al., 1990; D'Amour & Charbonneau, 1992; Smith et al., 1993; Goerz et al., 1994). This means that HCB is a mixed-type cytochrome-P-450-inducing compound, with phenobarbital-inducible and 3-methylcholanthrene-inducible properties. Enzyme induction has been observed at relatively low doses in some studies. For instance, in Wistar rats fed HCB in the diet for 14 days, the low-effect level for induction of microsomal liver enzyme was 50 mg HCB/kg feed (approximately 2.5 mg/kg body weight per day), and the no-effect level was 20 mg HCB/kg feed (approximately 1 mg/kg body weight per day) (den Tonkelaar & van Esch, 1974).

The effects produced by subchronic exposure to HCB are similar to those observed in short-term studies, but are generally evident at lower doses (Courtney, 1979; US EPA, 1985a; ATSDR, 1990, 1994). At relatively high doses (32 mg/kg body weight per day or more for periods from several weeks to 90 days), reported effects have included death, skin lesions, behavioural and neurological changes, reduced body weight gain, increased organ weights, and altered thyroid function and serum levels of thyroid hormones (the latter effect is discussed later in this section). At lower doses, hepatotoxic effects have been commonly reported, including histological alterations, the induction of a variety of hepatic microsomal enzymes and porphyria.

The porphyrinogenic effects of exposure to HCB have been extensively studied since the seminal reports of Ockner & Schmid (1961) and De Matteis et al. (1961). These and subsequent earlier works, many of them conducted at relatively high doses, have been summarized by Courtney (1979), and much of this research is not discussed in this report. Porphyria has been observed in several species of laboratory mammals, most often manifested as increased levels of porphyrins and/or porphyrin precursors in the liver, other tissues and excreta. This disturbance in haem synthesis is associated with the inhibition of uroporphyrinogen decarboxylase activity (this enzyme converts uroporphyrinogen III to coproporphyrinogen III), leading to the accumulation of uroporphyrin and other highly carboxylated porphyrins, and with the induction of ALA synthetase (the enzyme controlling the rate of haem synthesis) (ATSDR, 1994). There is a delay before exposed rats become porphyric, which appears to reflect the time for the animals to receive a sufficient cumulative dose of

HCB (Krishnan et al., 1991, 1992), as well as the time needed for the porphyrins to accumulate to the level of overt porphyria (Kennedy et al., 1986; Kennedy & Wigfield, 1990). Although in most studies porphyria has been associated with longer-term exposure to HCB, rats exposed to doses of 25-50 mg HCB/kg body weight per day for as little as several days had increased levels of hepatic and urinary porphyrins (Krishnan et al., 1991, 1992). In another study, hepatic levels of highly carboxylated porphyrins were elevated by a single exposure to 50 mg HCB/kg body weight, although the latter result was not accompanied by clinical porphyria (Kennedy & Wigfield, 1990).

HCB-induced porphyria has been extensively studied in rats, in which dietary or gavage exposure of various strains to between 2.5 and 15 mg HCB/kg body weight per day for periods of 8 to 15 weeks has caused hepatic porphyria, and, in some studies, increased levels of porphyrins in the kidney and spleen (Grant et al., 1975; Kuiper-Goodman et al., 1977; Goldstein et al., 1978; Mendoza et al., 1979; Rizzardini & Smith, 1982; Teschke et al., 1983; Smith et al., 1985b; Green et al., 1989; Van Ommen et al., 1989; Kennedy & Wigfield, 1990; Smith et al., 1990; Den Besten et al., 1993). A no-observed-effect-level (NOEL) for HCB-induced porphyria was not determined in these studies. Although the data on other species are limited, levels of hepatic or urinary porphyrins were increased in mice of various strains fed diets containing 200 mg HCB/kg feed (yielding approximate doses of 24 mg HCB/kg body weight per day) for periods of 7 to 15 weeks in some studies (Smith & Francis, 1983; Rizzardini et al., 1988; Vincent et al., 1989), and porphyria was induced in Japanese quail following short-term oral and intraperitoneal exposure to 500 mg HCB/kg body weight per day (section 9.1.2).

The lowest doses producing porphyrinogenic and other effects on the liver in a subchronic study were reported by den Tonkelaar et al. (1978). Groups of five pigs exposed for 90 days to doses of 0.5 mg/kg body weight per day or more in the diet had increased urinary levels of coproporphyrin and alterations in liver histology and microsomal enzyme activities, but no effects were observed at 0.05 mg/kg body weight per day. However, marked excretion of coproporphyrin alone is not a characteristic of the inhibition of uroporphyrinogen decarboxylase in animal systems.

Female rats are more sensitive than males to the porphyrinogenic effects of exposure to HCB. In various strains of rats exposed to doses of 5 to 10 mg HCB/kg body weight per day in the diet or by gavage, for periods of between 3 months or more, females developed a marked porphyria which was absent or much reduced in males (Grant et al., 1975; Kuiper-Goodman et al., 1977; Rizzardini & Smith, 1982; Smith et al., 1985b). In a number of studies, the basis for the susceptibility to HCB-induced porphyria of female rats compared to males has been examined. Grant et al. (1975) reported that ovariectomy decreased, and castration increased, the accumulation of porphyrins in the livers of female and male Sprague-Dawley rats with subchronic exposure to HCB, suggesting a role for steroid hormones in the development of porphyria in this species. In another study, female Fischer-344 rats with HCB-induced porphyria had higher levels of cytochrome P-450IA isoenzymes and ethoxyresorufin-*O*-deethylase activity than males, whereas males had higher levels of total cytochrome P-450 and activities of microsomal monooxygenases associated with cytochrome P-450IIB1 (Smith et al., 1990). In Fischer-344 rats with HCB-induced porphyria, sex-related differences in urinary and hepatic porphyrin levels were paralleled by differences in the excretion of phenolic metabolites, particularly pentachlorothiophenol (Rizzardini & Smith, 1982). These findings were further investigated in a short-term study by D'Amour & Charbonneau (1992), which indicated that male rats may be more resistant to HCB-induced porphyria than females because hepatic conjugation of HCB with glutathione is more important in males. Male Sprague-Dawley rats receiving a porphyrinogenic dose of HCB (100 mg HCB/kg body weight per day by gavage for 5 days) had significantly lower hepatic gluthione concentration and higher glutathione transferase activity (to 3,4-dichloronitrobenzene) than controls, whereas no significant differences were observed in females. Biliary excretion of PCTP (a metabolite of glutathione conjugation) and the rate of elimination of HCB from the liver were greater in males than in females.

Other mechanistic studies have suggested the involvement of oxidative metabolism of HCB in the development of porphyria, although the mechanism remains to be elucidated. In female Wistar rats co-treated with 300 mg HCB/kg in the diet (approximately 15 mg HCB/kg body weight per day) and triacetyloleandomycin (TAO) (to selectively inhibit cytochrome P-450IIIA1/2 and thereby prevent the oxidative biotransformation of HCB) for 10-13 weeks, both the excretion of PCP and TCHQ (tetrachlorohydroquinone, the reduced analogue of the reactive tetrachlorobenzoquinone) and the extent of hepatic porphyria and urinary porphyrin excretion were greatly diminished (Van Ommen et al., 1989; Den Besten et al., 1993). In 13-week feeding studies on female Wistar rats exposed to 300 mg HCB/kg diet (approximately 15 mg HCB/kg body weight per day) in the presence or absence of TAO, the degree of porphyria was better correlated with excretion of PCP than TCHQ, and in comparative studies pentachlorobenzene (which is metabolized to PCP by a different mechanism than for HCB) was not porphyrinogenic (Den Besten et al., 1993).

In addition, it has been suggested that the aryl hydrocarbon receptor (Ah receptor) may be involved in the accumulation of hepatic porphyrins in mice (Linko et al., 1986; Hahn et al., 1988, 1989). Ah-responsive strains of inbred mice were more sensitive to hepatic porphyrin accumulation after HCB exposure than non-responsive mice (Smith & Francis, 1983; Hahn et al., 1988), and HCB has been shown to be a weak agonist for the Ah receptor (Hahn et al., 1989).

Full discussion of the evidence for a unifying hypothesis of porphyria induced by HCB and other chemicals that act in a similar way, as well as for human sporadic porphyria cutanea tarda, is beyond the scope of this document. There is however, substantial experimental and human evidence implicating a complex interaction between hepatocellular iron and oxidative processes leading to the oxidation of unstable uroporphyrinogen to uroporphyrin, possibly mediated by induced cytochrome P-450 isozymes (reviewed by Smith & De Matteis, 1990). There is evidence that inhibition of uroporphyrinogen decarboxylase may occur through formation of an inhibitor of the enzyme during the oxidation of uroporphyrinogen (Rios de Molina et al., 1980; Smith & De Matteis, 1990). HCB may act partly through induction and uncoupling of the cytochrome P-450 system to form reactive oxygen species, especially in the presence of an increased available iron pool (Smith & De Matteis, 1990; Den Besten et al., 1993).

Subchronic exposure to low doses of HCB has also caused changes in calcium homoeostasis and bone morphometry. Male Fischer-344 rats administered HCB by gavage in corn oil had elevated serum levels of 1,25-dihydroxy-vitamin-D_3 and reduced calcium excretion after 5 weeks, and increased femur density, weight and strength after 15 weeks. These effects were evident at 0.7 mg/kg body weight per day but not at 0.07 mg/kg body weight per day (Andrews et al., 1989, 1990).

While technical HCB is known to be contaminated with chlorinated dibenzo-*p*-dioxins, dibenzofurans and biphenyls (Villanueva et al., 1974; Goldstein et al., 1978), the effects (primarily hepatic) of subchronic dietary exposure of rats to either pure or technical HCB were virtually identical, indicating that the effects observed in this study were due to the parent compound (Goldstein et al., 1978).

In a number of studies on various strains of rats, short-term or subchronic exposure to HCB affected the thyroid, as indicated by decreased serum levels of total and free thyroxine (T_4) and often, to a lesser extent, triiodothyronine (T_3). In some instances, these are accompanied by compensatory increases in thyroid weight, circulating levels of thyroid-stimulating hormone or iodine uptake by the thyroid (Rozman et al., 1986; Kleiman de Pisarev et al., 1989, 1990; Van Raaij et al., 1991a, 1993a, 1993b; Foster et al., 1993; Den Besten et al., 1993; Sopena de Krakoff et al., 1994). Den Besten et al. (1993) reported such effects in rats exposed to as little as 9.5 mg/kg body weight per day following dietary exposures for 13 weeks, although effect levels were somewhat higher in other studies, which involved exposure for a shorter duration and/or employed an aqueous vehicle. Somewhat different effects (decreased levels of T_3 in serum and no change in T_4, accompanied by increased uptake of iodine by the thyroid) were observed in hamsters exposed to 100-200 mg HCB/kg feed (approximately 12-24 mg/kg body weight per day) for 18-28 weeks (Smith et al., 1987).

The mechanisms that have been advanced to account for the effects of HCB on the thyroid include accelerated metabolism of thyroid hormones by HCB-induced enzymes or accelerated deiodination of thyroxine, in conjunction with increased biliary excretion (Kleiman de Pisarev, 1989; Van Raaij et al., 1993b), and interference with plasma transport of thyroid hormones through displacement of T_4 from binding sites on proteins (Van Raaij et al., 1991a, 1993a). Van Raaij et al. (1991b, 1993a) reported that intraperitoneal injection of pentachlorophenol and tetrachloro-hydroquinone, but not HCB itself, decreased serum thyroxine levels in rats, indicating that these metabolites may be involved in the effects of HCB on the thyroid. These authors reported that PCP was a more effective competitor for thyroxine-binding sites of serum carriers *in vitro*, and more effective at occupying carrier sites in *ex vivo* experiments, than HCB (van Raaij et al., 1991a), and demonstrated that T_4 binding sites were partially occupied in the serum of rats exposed to HCB (Van Raaij et al., 1993a). In the latter study, it was estimated that competition for thyroid hormone binding sites, by PCP metabolized from HCB, could account for almost half of the observed reduction in serum levels of T_4.

7.3 Long-term toxicity and carcinogenicity

A range of non-neoplastic effects from long-term exposure to HCB, which are primarily hepatotoxic, have been observed at relatively low doses. In a two-generation study with Sprague-Dawley rats, liver and heart weights were increased in F_0 males exposed to TWA doses of 0.29 and 1.50 mg/kg body weight per day in the diet for 3 months, and histopathological changes in the liver were observed in F_1 animals of both sexes exposed to maternal doses of 0.29-0.38 and 1.50-1.90 mg HCB/kg body weight per day in diet *in utero*, through nursing, and then continued on the same diet as their parents for their lifetimes. The no-effect level in this study was 0.06-0.07 mg/kg body weight per day (Arnold et al., 1985; Arnold & Krewski, 1988). Dietary exposures of Sprague-Dawley rats to 10 mg/kg and above (approximately 0.5-0.6 mg/kg body weight per day) for 9-10 months induced *in vivo* mixed-function oxidase activity, as indicated by reductions in drug-induced sleeping times (Grant et al., 1974). Exposure of Sprague-Dawley rats to 5 mg HCB/kg in diet (approximately 0.25-0.30 mg/kg body weight per day) for 3-12 months caused proliferation of smooth endoplasmic reticulum, altered mitochondria and increased numbers of storage vesicles in liver, but these effects were not evident at 1 mg/kg in diet (approximately 0.05-0.06 mg/kg body weight per day) (Mollenhauer et al., 1975; 1976). In a study by Böger et al. (1979), oral administration of 2, 8 or 32 mg HCB to female Wistar rats twice weekly for 203 days (0.57, 2.3 or 9.1 mg HCB/kg body weight per day) resulted in hepatocellular enlargement, proliferated smooth endoplasmic reticulum, increased glycogen and porphyrin deposits, and enlarged mitochondria, but these effects were not seen at a lower dose (0.5 mg HCB/kg body weight twice weekly, or 0.14 mg HCB/kg body weight per day). Bleavins et al. (1984a) reported that exposure of female mink to a dietary concentration of 1 mg/kg (estimated to yield a dose of 0.16 mg/kg body weight per day) for 47 weeks significantly increased serotonin concentrations in the hypothalamus of dams, and depressed hypothalamic dopamine concentrations in kits exposed *in utero* and through nursing.

As in subchronic studies, female rats were more sensitive than males to porphyria induced by chronic exposure to HCB. Grant et al. (1974) reported that in Sprague-Dawley rats fed diets containing HCB for 9-10 months, reduced weight gain and porphyria were observed in females, but not males, receiving 80 or 160 mg HCB/kg feed (approximately 4 or 8 mg HCB/kg body weight per day). A dose-related increase in relative liver weights and in the hepatic content of HCB was noted in both sexes. Hepatic enzyme activities and cytochrome P-450 activities were increased in males administered 40 mg HCB/kg feed or more. Exposure to 10 mg HCB/kg feed (approximately 0.5-0.6 mg HCB/kg body weight per day) induced *in vivo* mixed-function oxidase activity, as indicated by reductions in sleeping time for pentobarbital and zoxazolamine exposure.

The carcinogenicity of HCB has been assessed in several bioassays in rats, mice and hamsters. The following discussion is limited principally to the four studies in which adequate numbers of animals of both sexes were exposed for a sufficient length of time to more than one dose level.

Cabral et al. (1977) and Cabral & Shubik (1986) reported a statistically significant increase of liver cell tumours (hepatomas) in groups of 30-60 male and female Syrian golden hamsters fed 50, 100 or 200 mg HCB/kg (4, 8 or 16 mg/kg body weight per day) HCB in their diets for life. The incidence of "haemangioendotheliomas" of the liver was significantly increased in both sexes at 200 mg/kg and in males at 100 mg/kg, and of alveolar adenomas of the thyroid in males at 200 mg/kg. (The latter finding is interesting in the light of reports of excesses of thyroid neoplasms, or of enlargement of the thyroid, in human populations with elevated exposures to HCB (section 8.1.)) The authors reported that three of the hepatic "haemangioendotheliomas" (which are non-invasive by definition) metastasized. It seems likely, therefore, that these tumours were malignant, though misclassified.

In another study, HCB was administered in the diet to groups of 30 or 50 outbred male and female Swiss mice at concentrations of 0, 50, 100 and 200 mg/kg (0, 6, 12 and 24 mg/kg body weight per day) for 120 weeks (Cabral et al., 1979; Cabral & Shubik, 1986). In females exposed to 200 mg/kg, a statistically significant increase in the incidence of "liver cell tumours (hepatomas)" was noted. "Hepatomas" were also elevated, though not significantly, in males at this dose and in both sexes at 100 mg/kg. The number of tumour-bearing animals, the latent period, and the multiplicity and size of tumours increased with dose.

Arnold et al. (1985) and Arnold & Krewski (1988) investigated the potential carcinogenicity to rats of combined *in utero*, lactational and oral exposure to analytical grade HCB. Groups of 40 or more weanling male and female Sprague-Dawley rats were fed diets containing 0, 0.32, 1.6, 8 or 40 mg HCB/kg. (Based on data supplied by the author, mean doses for males were 0, 0.01, 0.06, 0.29 and 1.50 mg/kg body weight per day and for females 0, 0.01, 0.07, 0.38 and 1.90 mg/kg body weight per day). After 3 months, the F_0 rats were bred, and 50 F_1 pups of each sex were randomly selected from each group. From weaning, the F_1 animals were continued on the same diet for their lifetimes (up to 130 weeks). In exposed F_1 females, increased incidences of neoplastic liver nodules and adrenal phaeochromocytomas were noted at the highest dose. A significantly increased incidence of parathyroid adenomas was noted in males receiving 40 mg HCB/kg in their diet.

In a study by Lambrecht et al. (1983a,b; Ertürk et al., 1986), groups of 94 weanling Sprague-Dawley rats were fed diets containing 0, 75 or 150 mg/kg (4 and 8 mg/kg body weight per day for males and 5 and 9 mg/kg body weight per day for females, respectively) for up to 2 years. Statistically significant increases in the incidence of hepatomas/haemangiomas and of renal cell adenomas were noted at both doses in animals of both sexes surviving beyond 12 months. Incidences of hepatocellular carcinomas and bile duct adenomas/carcinomas were also elevated in females at both doses. In female rats, significant increases in the incidences of adrenal cortical adenomas at 75 mg/kg and phaeochromocytomas at both doses were reported. Lambrecht et al. (1983b) reported a leukaemia involving the thymus, spleen, liver and kidney in rats exposed to HCB in this study, but did not present any quantitative data. The results of this study were only reported in summary form, with few details of the study protocol and results. In addition, HCB was incorporated into the diet as a powder in this study, raising the possibility that some of the effects observed may have been in part attributable to the inhalation of aerosolized HCB.

High incidences of liver tumours have also been reported in some more limited studies in which single dietary concentrations (100 or 200 mg/kg) were administered to small groups (i.e., between 4 and 15) of females of three strains of rats (Smith & Cabral, 1980; Smith et al., 1985b); in one strain (Fischer-344), hepatocellular carcinomas were observed (Smith et al., 1985b). HCB has not, however, been carcinogenic in several other studies in various strains of mice (Theiss et al., 1977; Shirai et al., 1978; Smith et al., 1989), perhaps as a result of the low doses, short durations of exposure and/or small group sizes employed. Results were also negative in a second study by Arnold et al. (1985), in which groups of 50 male Sprague-Dawley rats were fed diets containing 40 mg HCB/kg in conjunction with various levels of vitamin A for 119 weeks, indicating the probable higher sensitivity of the two-generation carcinogenesis bioassay.

Ertürk et al. (1982, 1986; Lambrecht et al., 1982a,b) examined the tumorigenic activity of subchronic exposure to HCB in both sexes of Swiss mice, Syrian golden hamsters and Sprague-Dawley rats at dietary levels of 0, 100 and 200 mg/kg (mice) and 0, 200 and 400 mg/kg (hamsters and rats) for 90 days. At day 91, 25 of 50 animals in each group were sacrificed for histological examination, with the remainder being sacrificed at 6-week intervals (up to 341, 361 and 424 days for mice, hamsters and rats, respectively). The results of these studies were reported in summary form only, and much of the quantitative data were not presented. The authors reported that, as the experiment progressed, treated animals developed hepatomas, bile duct adenomas, renal adenomas and carcinomas, and lymphosarcomas of the thymus, spleen, and lymph nodes. However, the only tumour and species for which they presented clear evidence of a treatment-related increase in incidence was for lymphatic tumours in mice (Ertürk et al., 1982). Lymphatic and renal neoplasms were observed as early as the end of the 90-day period. It is not clear from these reports which tumours each species developed or the dietary levels associated with the observed effects, as well as other experimental details.

Results from a number of studies have indicated that HCB is a co-carcinogen or promoter of cancer. Concomitant exposure to 50 mg HCB/kg in diet (approximately 6 mg HCB/kg body weight per day) enhanced the induction of liver tumours by polychlorinated terphenyl (at 250 mg/kg diet) in male ICR mice (Shirai et al., 1978). Exposure to HCB (100-200 mg/kg in diet (approximately 5-10 mg HCB/kg body weight per day) or 1 mmole/kg i.p. at 1 and 5 weeks) promoted the development of hepatocellular carcinomas and/or hepatic gamma-glutamyltranspeptidase-positive foci initiated by diethylnitrosamine in various strains of rats (Pereira et al., 1982; Herren-Freund & Pereira, 1986; Stewart et al., 1989).

In some recent studies, the possible mechanisms by which HCB induces tumours in animals have been investigated.

Bouthillier et al. (1991) presented the results of studies of Sprague-Dawley rats exposed to 100 mg HCB/kg by gavage for periods of several weeks, which indicated that the observed increase in renal tumours in male Sprague-Dawley rats following exposure to HCB (Lambrecht et al., 1983b; Ertürk et al., 1986) is related to protein droplet nephropathy. The mechanism by which structurally diverse hydrocarbons induce hyaline droplet nephropathy in male rats has been well documented and involves accumulation of alpha-2u-globulin, resulting in necrosis, regeneration and, in some cases, tumours. This response is sex- and species-specific, and hence is unlikely to be relevant to humans. This mechanism does not, however, explain the increased (but lower) incidence of renal tumours in females also reported by Lambrecht et al. (1983b).

Carthew & Smith (1994) hypothesized that some HCB-induced hepatic tumours in rats may be produced by a non-genotoxic mechanism. They noted that hepatotoxicity of HCB in rodents gives rise to peliosis and necrosis with haemosiderosis, indicating that vascular damage has occurred, and confirmed the presence of such damage in the liver of chronically HCB-exposed rats by the identification of widespread fibrin deposits, using an antibody to rat fibrin. These deposits occurred in association with abundant haemosiderosis in hepatocytes and areas of widened hepatic sinusoids. On this basis, it was suggested that the formation of hepatomas and haemangiomas with elements of peliosis could be the result of compensatory hyperplastic responses to hepatocellular necrosis and the simultaneous loss of hepatocellular cords, perhaps potentiated by the accumulation of iron in the liver.

Mechanistic studies that address the relevance to humans of the remaining tumour types induced in rodents by HCB have not been identified.

7.4 Mutagenicity and related end-points

HCB has not been found to be genotoxic in most studies conducted to date. HCB did not cause either frameshift or base pair substitution mutations in *Salmonella typhimurium* at doses of as much as 10 mg/plate with or without metabolic activation, with both rat and hamster liver activation systems, pre-incubation and plate incorporation methods, and technical and 99.9% pure HCB (Haworth et al., 1983; Górski et al., 1986; Siekel et al., 1991). A weak positive response in *S. typhimurium* strain TA98 at 50 and 100 μg/plate was reported by Gopalaswamy & Aiyar (1986) and Gopalaswamy & Nair (1992). However, the authors also reported mutagenic activity for lindane, in contrast to the results of other studies (e.g., Haworth et al., 1983). Doses of up to 1000 μg/plate of HCB did not induce tryptophan reversion or DNA damage in *Escherichia coli* strains WP2 and WP2uvrA with or without metabolic activation (Siekel et al., 1991).

There have been reports of mutagenic activity for HCB in eukaryotic cells *in vitro*, although these studies have limitations. Guerzoni et al. (1976) reported a positive finding for methionine reversion in *Saccharomyces cerevisiae* strain 632/4 exposed to HCB, but Brusick (1986) did not consider the observed increase to meet current standards of a positive response. In addition, only a single dose level was used in that study, and there was no exogenous metabolic activation. Kuroda (1986) reported that in cultured Chinese hamster lung cells (V79), HCB did not induce OUA^r mutations, but did induce $8AG^r$ mutations. However, both the magnitude of the increase (which was small, roughly $1/10^5$ survivors at the two highest doses) and uncertain dose-response indicate that this response is open to question.

Oral administration of as much as 221 mg HCB/kg body weight per day to male rats for 5 or 10 days failed to induce dominant lethal effects in two different studies (Khera, 1974; Simon et al., 1979), although Simon et al. (1979) did observe a slight reduction in male reproductive performance (numbers of females inseminated and impregnated). Rumsby et al. (1992) reported that liver neoplasms that developed in iron-overloaded C57Bl/10ScSn mice exposed for 18 months to 0.01% HCB in the diet were not associated with a high frequency of mutations in the Ha-ras proto-oncogene at codon 61. Only two mutations were observed at different sites, from 23 preneoplastic and neoplastic lesions examined, indicating that activation of the Ha-ras gene is not an important event in the hepatocarcinogenicity of HCB in this test system.

HCB has not been found to be clastogenic in the few available studies in which this end-point has been examined. The compound did not increase the frequency of sister chromatid exchanges in the bone marrow of male mice given as much as 400 mg/kg body weight (by an unspecified route), although the lack of detail in reporting the test protocol and results limits the interpretation of this study (Górski et al., 1986). HCB did not induce chromosomal aberrations *in vitro* in cultured Chinese hamster fibroblast cells at concentrations as high as 12 mg/ml, with or without metabolic activation (Ishidate, 1988), or in human peripheral blood lymphocytes exposed to up to 0.1 mmol/litre (Siekel et al., 1991). Treatment of rats with 1000 mg HCB/kg diet for 15 days was hepatotoxic, but did not cause early diploidization in hepatocytes as measured by flow cytometry (Rizzardini et al., 1990).

The results of less specific assays also indicate that HCB does not interact strongly with DNA, although there are two reports that the compound binds, at low levels, to DNA. After incubating hepatocytes isolated from phenobarbital-treated rats with ^{14}C-HCB (5 μM) for 20 h, Stewart & Smith (1987) reported the maximum amount of radioactivity associated with DNA was < 9.9×10^{-5}% of the substrate added, and was only marginally above that of hepatocytes held at 4 °C; the authors considered this to be significantly lower than expected for hepatocarcinogens. Gopalaswamy & Nair (1992) also reported a low order of binding of HCB to DNA from the livers of rats exposed to 25 mg HCB/kg. Short-term exposure (<1 day) of rats to oral doses of 700 or 1400 mg/kg body weight (Kitchin & Brown, 1989) or to as much at 300 mg/kg body weight i.p. (Górski et al., 1986) did not cause hepatic DNA damage, as measured by alkaline elution.

7.5 Reproductive and developmental toxicity

Relatively low doses of HCB have been found to affect some reproductive tissues in female monkeys. Oral exposure of cynomolgus monkeys to 0.1 mg/kg body weight per day in gelatin capsules for 90 days caused stratification of the ovarian germinal epithelium (Babineau et al., 1991; Jarrell et al., 1993a). Higher dosages (1.0 and 10.0 mg/kg body weight per day) were associated with cellular degeneration of this surface epithelium. The low dosage was associated with ultrastructural as well as light microscopic changes in surface epithelium (Babineau et al., 1991; Sims et al., 1991).

In ovarian follicles the low dose was associated with an increased number of lysosomal elements in germ cells (Singh et al., 1990a). The basal lamina was thickened. Higher dosages were associated with greater degenerative changes in their cells and granulosa cells (Singh et al., 1991, 1990b).

These studies demonstrated changes in ovarian tissues with no other evidence of toxicity. In particular, the induction of superovulation with human menopausal gondotrophin (HMG) in these animals was associated with a normal estradiol response, oocyte recovery, oocyte maturation, *in vitro* fertilization and early embryo development (Jarrell et al., 1993a). These studies confirm the findings of Iatropoulous et al. (1976) in which the administration of 8 to 128 mg/kg body weight (by gavage in 1% methylcellulose) for 60 days induced severe follicular degeneration in primordial germ cells, pseudostratification of the ovarian surface epithelium, hepatic degeneration and severe systemic toxicity in Rhesus monkeys.

In subsequent studies of similarly treated animals, the higher doses were associated with reduced luteal phase progesterone and blunted estradiol responses to HMG (Foster et al., 1992a,b). Reduction in adrenal steroidogenesis occurred in ovariectomized rats in response to exposure to HCB at concentrations of 1, 10 and 100 mg/kg body weight for 30 days (Foster et al., 1995).

In contrast, the results of studies on a variety of species have indicated that repeated exposure to HCB can affect male reproduction, but only at relatively high doses. Mice exposed to 250 mg HCB per kg feed (approximately 30 mg HCB/kg body weight per day) for 21 days had reduced serum testosterone levels; based on the results of *in vitro* tests, it was suggested that this was due to increased metabolism by hepatic microsomal enzymes induced by HCB (Elissalde & Clark, 1979). Histological changes in the testes (retarded sexual maturation) were noted in pigs fed a diet yielding a dose of 50 mg HCB/kg body weight per day for 90 days (den Tonkelaar et al., 1978). The mating index for male rats receiving five consecutive daily gavage doses of 221 mg HCB/kg body weight in corn oil was decreased compared to those receiving 0 or 70 mg/kg body weight However, the fertility index for the mated female rats (sperm positive smears) was not affected (Simon et al., 1979).

As discussed in the following paragraphs, placental and lactational transfer of HCB, demonstrated in a number of species, can adversely affect both the fetus and nursing offspring. The lactational route appears to be more important than placental transfer. Adverse effects on suckling infants are generally observed more frequently, and at lower doses, than are embryotoxic or fetotoxic effects.

Grant et al. (1977) conducted a four-generation study on female (20/dose level) and male (10/dose level) weanling Sprague-Dawley rats fed diets containing 0, 10, 20, 40, 80, 160, 320 or 640 mg HCB/kg feed. The two highest doses caused some deaths in the F_0 dams before first whelping, and reduced the fertility index. Dietary levels of 160 mg/kg or more reduced litter sizes, increased the number of stillbirths, and adversely affected pup survival. Similar effects were seen at 80 mg/kg after the first two generations, while 40 mg/kg was hepatotoxic to the F_{1a} and F_{3a} pups. A dietary level of 20 mg/kg (approximately 1-1.2 mg/kg body weight per day) was designated as the no-observed-effect level.

Arnold et al. (1985) fed groups of male and female Sprague-Dawley rats from weaning on diets containing up to 40 mg HCB/kg. The rats were then bred at 3 months, and the F_1 pups were continued on the same diet for their lifetimes. HCB had no effect on fertility, but pup survival was significantly reduced in the 40 mg/kg group (calculated doses of 1.50 and 1.90 mg/kg body weight per day for males and females, respectively).

In other studies, maternal doses in the range from 1.4 to 4 mg/kg given to rats and cats have been found to be hepatotoxic and/or affected the survival or growth of nursing offspring. In some cases, these or higher doses reduced litter sizes and/or increased numbers of stillbirths (Mendoza et al., 1977, 1978, 1979; Hansen et al., 1979; Kitchin et al., 1982).

Mink are particularly sensitive to the effects of prenatal and perinatal exposure to HCB; the offspring of mink fed diets containing concentrations as low as 1 mg/kg (approximately 0.16 mg/kg body weight per day) for 47 weeks (prior to mating and throughout gestation and nursing) had reduced birth weights and increased mortality (Rush et al., 1983; Bleavins et al., 1984b).

The available data on the developmental toxicity of HCB are limited. CD-1 mice administered 100 mg/kg body weight by gavage on days 7-16 of gestation had a significantly increased incidence of abnormal fetuses per litter, and one case of renal agenesis was reported. Some cleft palates were produced, but they all occurred in one litter. This dose also increased maternal liver-to-body weight ratios and decreased fetal body weights (Courtney et al., 1976). In a series of studies reported by Andrews & Courtney (1986), combined *in utero* and lactational exposure of CD-1 mice and CD rats (strain unclear, probably Sprague-Dawley) to HCB (mouse dams received 10 or 50 mg/kg body weight per day, and rats 10 mg/kg body weight per day, by gavage during gestation) resulted in increases in body weight and kidney weights of pups of both species, along with enlarged kidneys and a few cases of hydronephrosis. Increased liver weights were observed in rat pups, and the occurrence of abnormal kidneys was sporadic, with no dose-response relationship in studies with mice. Khera (1974) reported a significant increase in the incidence of unilateral or bilateral 14th rib in litters of Wistar rats receiving doses of 80 and 120 mg HCB/kg body weight during gestation, but maternal toxicity (loss of body weight and neurological effects) and reduced fetal weights were noted in animals in these groups. (It should be noted that, based on the biological half-lives reported for HCB in mammals (section 6.2), the concentration of HCB in the dams in these studies would not have reached the maximum that might occur as a result of intake over a longer period).

Neurobehavioural development was affected in the offspring of rats exposed to 2.5 or 25 mg/kg body weight per day by gavage 2 weeks prior to breeding. Pups in both treated groups were hyperactive (based on tests of negative geotaxic reflex, olfactory discrimination, and exploratory locomotor activity) at 6-20 days of age. Pups from the high treatment groups showed reduced acoustic startle response at 23 days of age, but a significantly increased response at 90 days. These doses did not affect learning (swim T-maze) or motor activity in older offspring, nor maternal or fetal body weights, length of gestation, number of pups/litter at birth, or number of days to eye opening (Goldey & Taylor, 1992).

Lilienthal et al. (1996) recently reported HCB-induced effects on neurobehavioural development of rat pups exposed both maternally and through the diet (dams were exposed to 0, 8 or 16 mg HCB/kg diet for 90 days prior to mating and throughout gestation and nursing, after which the offspring were fed the same levels for 150 days). Exposure to HCB did not affect the mean body weight of the pups (except males at 150 days of age), or the number of pups/litter, but did increase the mean body weight of dam, and their liver-to-body weight ratios. Schedule-controlled behaviour was affected at 8 and 16 mg HCB/kg diet (0.64 and 1.28 mg/kg body weight per day), as indicated by a dose-related decrease in post-reinforcement pause at the end of the experiment. Exploratory locomotor activity, open field behaviour at 21 days of age, and active avoidance learning at 90 days of age were unaffected.

7.6 Immunotoxicity

The results of a number of studies have indicated that HCB affects the immune system, with immunosuppressive effects in mice and immunostimulatory effects in rats (summarized by Vos, 1986).

Balb/C mice exposed to 5 mg HCB/kg diet (approximately 0.6 mg/kg body weight per day) for 3 to 18 weeks were more susceptible to *Leishmania* infection (Loose, 1982) and had reductions in resistance to a challenge with tumour cells and in the cytotoxic macrophage activity of the spleen (Loose et al., 1981). Barnett et al. (1987) reported that Balb/C mice exposed to maternal doses of 0.5 or 5 mg HCB/kg body weight per day *in utero* and through nursing had severe depression of the delayed-type hypersensitivity response to a contact allergen (oxazolone). In a number of studies, exposure of mice to diets containing 167 mg HCB/kg in diet (approximately 20 mg HCB/kg body weight per day) for several weeks depressed humoral immunity, cell-mediated immunity and host resistance (Vos, 1986; Carthew et al., 1990).

In rats or rhesus monkeys with oral exposure to between 3 and 120 mg HCB/kg body weight per day for periods from 3 weeks to 6 months in various studies, proliferative histopathological effects in the thymus, spleen, lymph nodes, and/or lymphoid tissues of the lung have been observed (Kimbrough & Linder, 1974; Iatropoulos et al., 1976; Goldstein et al., 1978; Vos et al., 1979a,b; Kitchin et al., 1982). Gralla et al. (1977) observed that long-term exposure to 1 mg HCB/day (equivalent to a dose at the start of the experiment of roughly 0.12 mg/kg body weight per day) caused nodular hyperplasia of the gastric lymphoid tissue in beagle dogs.

In rats, prominent changes following dietary exposure to HCB include elevated IgM levels and an increase in the weights of the spleen and lymph nodes. Histopathologically, the spleen shows hyperplasia of B-lymphocytes in the marginal zone and follicles, while lymph nodes show an increase in proportions of high endothelial venules, indicative of activation. High endothelial-like venules are induced in the lung, as are accumulations of macrophages. Functional tests revealed an increase in cell-mediated immunity, as measured by DTH reactions, a notable increase in primary and secondary antibody response to tetanus toxoid, and decreased NK activity in the lung (Vos et al., 1979a,b). Stimulation of humoral and cell-mediated immunity occurred even at dietary levels as low as 4 mg HCB/kg (approximately 0.2 mg HCB/kg body weight per day); at such a dose conventional parameters for hepatotoxicity were unaltered (Vos et al., 1983). Therefore, the developing immune system of the rat seems to be particularly vulnerable to the immunotoxic action of HCB.

More recent studies indicate that HCB may cause autoimmune-like effects in the rat. Wistar rats treated with HCB had elevated levels of IgM, but not IgG, against the autoantigens single-stranded DNA, native DNA, rat IgG (representing rheumatoid factor), and bromelain-treated mouse erythrocytes (that expose phosphatidylcholine as a major autoantigen). It has been suggested that HCB activates a recently described B cell subset committed to the production of these antibodies (Schielen et al., 1993). The role of these autoantibodies is still a matter of controversy. Increased levels have been associated with various systemic autoimmune diseases, but a protective role of these autoantibodies against development of autoimmune disease has been postulated as well. Interesting in this respect are the observations that HCB had quite opposite effects in two different models of autoimmune disease in the Lewis rat. HCB treatment severely potentiates allergic encephalitis elicited by immunization with myelin in complete Freund's adjuvant, while it strongly inhibits the development of arthritic lesions elicited by complete Freund's adjuvant as such (Van Loveren et al., 1990).

A possible relation between the immunomodulatory properties of HCB and HCB-induced skin lesions, attributed in the literature to the porphyrinogenic action of HCB, was recently indicated. In rats treated with a combination of HCB and triacetyloleandomycin (TAO, a selective inhibitor of cytochrome P-450IIIa), porphyria was greatly reduced. Remarkably, combined treatment with HCB and TAO did not substantially affect the incidence and severity of skin lesions. In addition, TAO did not influence the immunomodulatory effect of HCB, including the formation of antibodies. From these findings it has been suggested that an immunological component underlies, at least in part, the HCB-induced skin lesions in the rat (Schielen et al., 1995).

8. EFFECTS ON HUMANS

8.1 General population exposure

Numerous reviews have been published of an accidental poisoning incident in Turkey that occurred in 1955-1959 as a result of HCB-treated wheat grain (distributed by the Turkish government for planting purposes) being ground into flour and made into bread (Schmid, 1960; Cam & Nigogosyan, 1963; Dogramaci, 1964; Peters, 1976; Courtney, 1979; Peters et al., 1982; US EPA, 1985a; Gocmen et al., 1989). In this incident, more than 600 cases of porphyria cutanea tarda (PCT) were clinically identified, and it was estimated that as many as 3000-5000 persons were affected, with a mortality of 10%. The condition developed primarily in children 4-14 years of age (roughly 80% of cases), occurring infrequently in adults and rarely in children under 4 years of age. In a number of reports, it has been suggested that males developed the condition in higher proportion than females. However, Dogramaci et al. (1962) demonstrated that the sex ratio was skewed in favour of males in both the affected and unaffected populations. In addition to disturbances in porphyrin metabolism (excretion of porphyrins and porphyrin precursors was greatly increased), clinical manifestations included skin lesions (erythema, bullae), ulcerations and resultant scarring, friable skin, hyperpigmentation, hypertrichosis, enlarged liver, weight loss, enlargement of the thyroid gland and lymph nodes, neurological effects, and a characteristic port wine colour of the urine (from increased excretion of porphyrins). In roughly half the cases, osteoporosis of extremities, deformation of the fingers or arthritis was also noted. The dermatological lesions, which occurred on the exposed parts of the body, particularly the face and hands, were often precipitated by sunlight. They tended to remit in winter and relapse during the spring and summer (Peters, 1976; Peters et al., 1982). The estimated dose was 50-200 mg/day for a number of months before manifestations of the disease became apparent (Cam & Nigogosyan, 1963); the basis for this estimate was not presented, however, making exposure calculations unreliable for this population. In 20- to 30-year follow-ups of exposed individuals, neurological, dermatological and orthopaedic abnormalities persisted, and there were elevated levels of porphyrins in excreta of some individuals (Peters et al., 1982; Peters et al., 1986; Gocmen et al., 1989).

In this incident, a disorder called "pembe yara" or "pink sore" was described in infants of mothers who either had PCT or had eaten HCB-contaminated bread. These infants developed characteristic pink cutaneous lesions, and often had fevers, diarrhea, vomiting, weakness, convulsions, enlarged livers and progressive wasting. It is noteworthy that PCT was not observed in these children (Cam, 1960; Peters et al., 1982). At least 95% of these children died within a year of birth, and in many villages no children between the ages of 2-5 years survived during the period 1955-1960. Elevated concentrations of HCB (levels were not quantified at the time, but the average concentration in milk from 56 porphyric mothers, 20-30 years after the incident, was 510 ng/g on a fat basis) were found in the mothers' milk and cessation of breast-feeding slowed the deterioration of infants with this disorder (Peters et al., 1966; Gocmen et al., 1989).

No adequate epidemiological studies of cancer in populations exposed to HCB in the environment were found in the literature. In long-term follow-up of the Turkish poisoning victims with porphyria (Peters et al., 1982; Cripps et al., 1984; Gocmen et al., 1989) there was no evidence of increased cancer incidence, although these studies were not designed to evaluate this end-point, and only a small fraction of the exposed people was followed up. There was a high frequency of enlarged thyroids in the Turkish poisoning victims (27% of men and 60% of women, compared to an average of 5% in the area (Peters et al., 1982)), but Gocmen et al. (1989) reported that they observed no malignant tumours of the liver or thyroid in 252 of the poisoning victims. In three patients who underwent thyroidectomy, histopathological examination indicated that the enlargement was due to colloidal goitre.

Grimalt et al. (1994) reported a small ecological study of cancer incidence (129 cases in all) in the inhabitants of a village in Spain located near a chlorinated solvents factory. There were statistically significant excesses of thyroid neoplasms and soft-tissue sarcomas in males, compared with the province as a whole, although these were based on only 2 and 3 cases, respectively. The exposures experienced by this population were somewhat unclear. Levels of HCB in ambient air and in the sera of volunteers were much higher in the village than in Barcelona (means of 35 ng/m^3 versus 0.3 ng/m^3 and 26 µg/litre versus 4.8 µg/litre, respectively), but the authors presented evidence that historical exposures had been much higher and indicated that all of the males with cancer for whom there were occupational histories had worked in the factory. Ambient air monitoring revealed that there were exposures to a variety of other compounds, including polychlorinated biphenyls, p,p'DDE, chloroform, carbon tetrachloride, trichloroethylene and tetrachloroethylene, but at similar or lower levels than in the reference community.

8.2 Occupational exposure

There have been case reports of workers developing PCT as a result of direct contact with HCB (Courtney, 1979; Currier et al., 1980), although there was no association between exposure to HCB and PCT in three cross-sectional studies of very small populations of exposed workers (Morley et al., 1973; Burns et al., 1974; Currier et al., 1980). There was no evidence of cutaneous porphyria in a cross-sectional study of the general population in Louisiana, USA, exposed to HCB through the improper transport and disposal of hex waste; however, plasma concentrations of HCB were significantly correlated with levels of coproporphyrin in urine and of lactic dehydrogenase in blood (Burns & Miller, 1975).

Available epidemiological studies on the carcinogenicity of HCB in occupationally exposed humans are restricted to one study of a cohort of 2391 magnesium metal production workers in Norway. Although the incidence of lung cancer was significantly elevated compared to that of the general population, workers were exposed to numerous other agents in addition to HCB, including coal tar, asbestos and dust of metal oxides and chlorides (Heldaas et al., 1989). Selden et al. (1989) reported a case of hepatocellular carcinoma in a 65-year-old man who had been employed for 26 years in an aluminum smelting plant, where he had potential exposure to a range of substances, including HCB, other chlorobenzenes, chlorophenols, dioxins and furans.

9. EFFECTS ON OTHER ORGANISMS IN THE LABORATORY AND FIELD

Data on the acute and chronic ecotoxicity of HCB are available for species from a number of trophic levels, including protozoans, algae, invertebrates and fish, for both the freshwater and marine environments. With reference to terrestrial organisms, toxicity data are available only for birds and mammals (the results of studies in mammals are summarized in chapter 7). Since HCB is nearly insoluble in water, and tends to partition from water to the atmosphere, the substance is lost rapidly from open-test solutions. Hence, it is difficult to maintain test concentrations for a sufficient time to establish concentration-effects profiles for aquatic organisms. Furthermore, HCB tends to bind to suspended solids in the water column and thus may not be bioavailable to test organisms. This discussion of the toxicity of HCB to aquatic organisms will therefore focus on tests conducted under flow-through conditions, static renewal conditions, or using closed vessels with minimal headspace. In addition, no consideration has been given to tests in which concentrations of HCB were well above its solubility in water (5 µg/litre at 25 °C).

9.1 Short-term exposure

9.1.1 Aquatic biota

Of four freshwater algal species tested, only one, *Chlorella pyrenoidosa*, was affected by concentrations of HCB in water at or below its limit of aqueous solubility. Reduced production of chlorophyll, dry matter, carbohydrate and nitrogen was observed for *C. pyrenoidosa* after exposure to a nominal concentration of 1 µg/litre HCB for 46 h in a static-closed system (Geike & Parasher, 1976a). A no-observed-effect concentration (NOEC) was not determined in this study.

At concentrations equal to its aqueous solubility in water (5 µg/litre), HCB was not lethal to the freshwater water flea *Daphnia magna* in a flow-through test in which concentrations of HCB were measured (Nebecker et al., 1989). In 96-h flow-through tests on marine invertebrates, exposure to HCB caused 13% mortality in pink shrimp (*Penaeus duorarum*) at a measured concentration of 7 µg HCB/litre, and 10% mortality in grass shrimp (*Palaemonetes pugio*) at 17 µg/litre. The NOEC values in these species were 2.3 µg/litre and 6.1 µg/litre, respectively (Parrish et al., 1974). In a static-closed system, there was a 10% reduction in reproduction of the ciliate protozoan *Euplotes vannus* after exposure to a nominal concentration of 10 µg/litre HCB for 48 h (Persoone & Uyttersprot, 1975).

The available data on freshwater fish species indicated no harmful effects at concentrations at or near the limit of solubility of HCB in water during acute exposure (Call et al., 1983; Ahmad et al., 1984). In the only available study for marine fish species, there were no effects on mortality in sheepshead minnow (*Cyprinodon variegatus*) after flow-through exposure to a measured concentration of 13 µg/litre HCB for 96 h (Parrish et al., 1974).

Limited data are available concerning the toxic effects of HCB in sediment on freshwater and marine biota. In a 96-h sediment toxicity test on the marine shrimp, *Crangon septemspinosa*, no mortality was observed at the highest concentration of HCB tested, 300 µg/litre (McLeese & Metcalfe, 1980).

Several studies have confirmed that there is a relatively constant body residue associated with acute lethality in freshwater fish, invertebrates and algae exposed to mono-to-pentachlorobenzenes (McCarty et al., 1992a; Ikemoto et al., 1992). The acute LC_{50} critical body residue for chlorobenzenes is 2 µmol/g wet weight, or 569.6 µg/g wet weight for HCB, assuming that HCB has the same mode of action as the other chlorobenzenes (McCarty et al., 1992b).

9.1.2 Terrestrial biota

The LD_{50} for HCB in herring gull (*Larus argentatus*) embryos injected on day 4 and tallied on day 25 was 4.3 µg/g body weight (Boersma et al., 1986). At a dose of 1.5 µg/g body weight, there were significant reductions in embryonic weight. Five-day LC_{50} values (i.e., 5 days of HCB-containing diet followed by 3 days of untreated diet) were 617 µg/g diet for 10-day-old ring-necked pheasants (*Phasianus colchicus*) and > 5000 µg/g diet for 5-day-old mallards (*Anas platyrhynchos*) (Hill et al., 1975). Induction of porphyria has been observed in studies of Japanese quail following administration of 500 µg HCB/g body weight per day for between 5 and 10 days either in food or via intraperitoneal injection (Buhler & Carpenter, 1986; Lambrecht et al., 1988).

9.2 Long-term exposure

9.2.1 Aquatic biota

Growth of cultures of the alga *Chlorella pyrenoidosa* was increased by exposure for 3 months to a nominal concentration of 1 µg HCB/litre (Geike & Parasher, 1976b), while that of the protozoan *Tetrahymena pyriformis* was decreased after a 10-day exposure to the same concentration (Geike & Parasher, 1976b).

After exposure to 5 µg HCB/litre for 10 days in a static-renewal system, crayfish (*Procambarus clarki*) experienced damage to the hepatopancreas (Laseter et al., 1976). The fertility of *Daphnia magna* was reduced by 50% after exposure for 14 days to a measured concentration of 16 µg/litre HCB in a static-closed system (Calamari et al., 1983). Significantly increased mortality was observed in amphipods, *Gammarus lacustris*, exposed to a measured concentration of 3.3 µg HCB/litre for 28 days under flow-through conditions (Nebecker et al., 1989). However, the results of this study indicated a weak-dose response relationship. In two other flow-through studies, there were no effects on survival, growth or reproduction of the amphipod *Hyallela azteca* and the worm *Lumbriculus variegatus* at a measured concentration of 4.7 µg HCB/litre (Nebecker et al., 1989).

In several studies, fathead minnows (*Pimephales promelas*) and rainbow trout (*Oncorhynchus mykiss*) experienced no mortality or effects on growth after exposure to levels of HCB approaching its aqueous solubility (Ahmad et al., 1984; Carlson & Kosian, 1987; US EPA, 1988; Nebecker et al., 1989). However, Laseter et al. (1976) reported liver necrosis in large-mouth bass (*Micropterus salmoides*) after an exposure for 10 days to 3.5 µg HCB/litre under flow-through conditions.

Guidelines for the protection and management of aquatic sediment quality in Ontario, Canada (Persaud et al., 1991) have given a no-observed-effect level (NOEL), a lowest-observed-effect level and a severe-effect level for a variety of contaminants. The values given for HCB are 10 ng/g dry weight, 20 ng/g dry weight and 24 000 ng/g organic carbon. The partitioning approach was used to determine the lowest-observed-effect level, whereas the severe-effect level was more dependent on the screening level concentration approach. The limitation of both approaches is that they are unable to separate the biological effects that are due to a combination of contaminants; thus while ecotoxicological effects can be established, these cannot be attributed to any one chemical contaminant. This is a very serious limitation since virtually all sediments are contaminated with a wide variety of pollutants, and there is no indication that HCB was the dominant pollutant.

Quantitative structure-activity relationships (QSAR) were used to estimate the narcotic toxicity for 19 species to predict NOELs (Van Leeuwen et al., 1992). The NOELs for water, sediment and residues in biota were predicted only on the basis of the octanol/water partition coefficient and relative molecular mass. The QSAR-derived level for HCB in sediments was 5814 ng/g dry weight (20.4 nmol/g in the reference) for sediments with 5% total organic carbon content. The adjusted value for sediment with 1% total organic carbon content is 1163 ng/g. There is no experimental verification of these calculations. Thus, no firm evidence is available on the critical levels of HCB in sediments.

9.2.2 Terrestrial biota

In adult Japanese quail (*Coturnix japonica*) fed diets containing HCB for 90 days, mortality was increased at 100 µg HCB/g in diet, and hatchability of eggs was significantly reduced at 20 µg/g (Vos et al., 1971, 1972). At 5 µg/g, increased liver weight, slight liver damage and increased faecal excretion of coproporphyrin were observed. Eurasian kestrels (*Falco tinnunculus*) fed mice containing 200 µg HCB/g fresh body weight for 65 days had significant weight loss, ruffling of feathers, tremors, increased liver weight and decreased heart weight (Vos et al., 1972).

The available long-term toxicity data for mammals are discussed in section 7.

10. EVALUATION OF HUMAN HEALTH RISKS AND EFFECTS ON THE ENVIRONMENT

10.1 Evaluation of human health risks

10.1.1 Exposure

Based on estimates of mean exposure from various media (section 5.2), the general population is exposed to HCB principally in food (mean intakes for adults range from 0.0004 to 0.0028 µg/kg body weight per day). Intakes are estimated to be considerably less for ambient air (3.4×10^{-5} to 2.1×10^{-4} µg/kg body weight per day) and drinking-water (2.2×10^{-6} to 4.4×10^{-5} µg/kg body weight per day). Based on these intakes, it is estimated that the total average daily intake of HCB from food, air and drinking-water is between 0.0004 and 0.003 µg/kg body weight per day.

Data on levels of occupational exposure to HCB are limited but indicate that workers in some industries may be exposed to higher levels of HCB than the general population, particularly in the manufacture of chlorinated solvents, and in the manufacture and application of chlorinated pesticides contaminated with HCB. In some instances inappropriate manufacturing and waste management practices may expose nearby populations to higher levels of HCB than the general population. Exposures may also be elevated in some indigenous subsistence populations, particularly those that consume large quantities of food species near the top of the food chain.

Owing to the elimination of HCB in breast milk, mean intakes by nursing infants are estimated to range from < 0.018 to 5.1 µg/kg body weight per day in various countries (see section 5.2.4 and Table 8).

10.1.2 Health effects

Available data on the effects of HCB in humans are limited principally to those of people exposed in an accidental poisoning incident that occurred in Turkey between 1955 and 1959. More than 600 cases of porphyria cutanea tarda (PCT) were observed, and infants of exposed mothers experienced cutaneous lesions, clinical symptoms and high mortality. It has been estimated that victims were exposed to an estimated dose of 50-200 mg HCB/day for an undetermined, but extended, period of time. However, the basis of this estimate was not provided, making exposure calculations unreliable for this population. Studies of the carcinogenicity of HCB in humans are limited to two small epidemiological studies of cancer incidence in populations with poorly characterized exposure to HCB as well as to numerous other chemicals. No excesses of neoplasms have been reported in long-term follow-up studies of the people with porphyria in the incident in Turkey, but only a small fraction of the population was followed-up, and these studies were not designed specifically to assess neoplastic end-points.

Hence, the available data on humans are inadequate to serve as a basis for assessment of effects from exposure to HCB. The remainder of this evaluation is, therefore, based on studies in animals.

Based on the studies reviewed in section 7, the critical effects induced by HCB in experimental animals comprise both non-neoplastic and neoplastic effects.

With respect to non-neoplastic effects, repeated exposure to HCB has been found to cause a wide range of non-neoplastic effects in several species of animals, with similar lowest-observed-effect-levels (LOELs) and no-observed-effect-levels (NOELs) for a number of end-points (see Table 9). In these studies, effects reported have included those on the liver in pigs and rats, on calcium metabolism in rats, on ovarian histopathology in monkeys, on immune function in mice and rats, on neurotransmitter levels in the hypothalamus of mink, on postnatal survival in mink, and on neurobehavioural development in rats. The range over which the various effects have been observed is quite narrow; the lowest LOELs compiled in Table 9 range from 0.1 to 0.7 mg/kg body weight per day, while the lowest NOELs range from 0.05 to 0.07 mg/kg body weight per day.

Based on the induction of a variety of tumours in hamsters, rats and mice exposed by ingestion, there is sufficient evidence that HCB is carcinogenic in animals. The available evidence indicates that HCB has little or no genotoxic activity and is therefore unlikely to be a direct-acting (genotoxic) carcinogen. However, the Task Group noted that tumours, some of which were malignant, have been induced in multiple species, at multiple sites, in some instances at doses that

Table 9. No-observed-effect and lowest-observed-effect levels (NOELs and LOELs) in mammals exposed to HCB

Species	Effect	NOEL (mg/kg body weight per day)	LOEL (mg/kg body weight per day)	Reference
Mouse	Depressed delayed-type hypersensitivity response to oxazolone in mice exposed to HCB in peanut butter *in utero* (throughout gestation) and via nursing to 45 days of age (section 7.6)	-	0.5[a]	Barnett et al. (1987)
Mouse	Increased susceptibility to *Leishmania* infection, and reductions in resistance to a challenge with tumour cells and in the cytotoxic macrophage activity of the spleen in mice with subchronic exposure to HCB in diet (section 7.6)	-	0.6	Loose et al. (1981); Loose (1982)
Rat	Alterations in Ca metabolism (increased serum 1,25-dihydroxy-vitamin-D_3 levels, reduced Ca excretion, alterations in femur density, bone morphometry and strength), increased liver weights, with subchronic gavage exposure to HCB (section 7.2)	0.07	0.7	Andrews et al. (1989, 1990)

Table 9 (contd).

Rat	Increased cell-mediated and humoral immune function, intraalveolar macrophage accumulation, microsomal ethoxyresorufin-O-deethylase activity, in rats exposed to HCB *in utero*, via nursing and in the diet to 5 weeks of age (section 7.6)	-	0.2[a]	Vos et al. (1983)
Rat	Increased organ weights (heart, brain and liver) in F_0 males, compound-related histological changes in liver of both sexes of F_1 rats with long-term exposure to HCB in diet (section 7.3)	0.05-0.07	0.27-0.35	Arnold et al. (1985); Arnold & Krewski (1988)
Rat	Ultrastructural changes in livers (proliferation of SER, altered mitochrondria, increase in numbers of storage vesicles) of rats with long-term exposure to HCB in diet (section 7.3)	0.05-0.06	0.25-0.30	Mollenhauer et al. (1975, 1976)
Rat	Induction of *in vivo* mixed-function oxidase activity in rats with long-term exposure to HCB in diet (section 7.3)	-	0.5-0.6	Grant et al. (1974)
Rat	Dose-related decrease in the post-reinforcement pause (PRP) after schedule-controlled operant conditioning of rats exposed to HCB *in utero*, through nursing, and up to post-natal day 150	-	0.64	Lilienthal et al. (1996)

Table 9 (contd).

Species	Effect	NOEL (mg/kg body weight per day)	LOEL (mg/kg body weight per day)	Reference
Mink	Increased serotonin concentrations in hypothalamus of mink dams with long-term dietary exposure to HCB, decreased dopamine levels in hypothalamus, reduced birth weights, and increased mortality to weaning in mink kits with *in utero* plus lactational exposure to HCB (sections 7.3, 7.5)	-	0.16[a]	Rush et al. (1983); Bleavins et al. (1984a,b)
Dog	Nodular hyperplasia of gastric lymphoid tissue in beagles with long-term exposure to HCB in gelatin capsules (section 7.6)	-	0.12	Gralla et al. (1977)
Pig	Increased urinary coproporphyrin and microsomal liver enzyme activity in pigs with subchronic exposure to HCB in diet (section 7.2)	0.05	0.05	Den Tonkelaar et al. (1978)

[a] Doses reported are those received by dams

were not overtly toxic in other respects and that are within an order of magnitude of those that produce more subtle toxicological effects, or following subchronic exposure. Although there is some evidence to suggest that HCB may cause cancer by indirect mechanisms, the evidence is not definitive at this time and does not address all tumour sites.

10.1.3 Approaches to risk assessment

The following is provided as a potential basis for derivation of guidance values. Since ingestion is by far the principal route of exposure and since the toxicological data for other routes of administration are insufficient for evaluation, only the oral route is addressed here, though the ultimate objective should be reduction of total exposure from all routes.

Based on the scientific evaluation of the data for the non-neoplastic and neoplastic end-points, two possible approaches to develop health-based guidance values were suggested.

.1.3.1 Non-neoplastic effects

The approach for non-neoplastic effects assumes a threshold for these effects and is based on the use of the NOAEL or NOEL and an uncertainty factor that takes account of interspecies and interindividual variation in sensitivity to the substance, as well as the quality of the available studies and the severity of effect.

The available data are sufficient to develop a Tolerable Daily Intake (TDI) for HCB. The lowest reported NOELs and LOELs for several different types of effects, such as those on the liver in rats and pigs, calcium metabolism in rats, ovarian morphology in monkeys, immune function in rats and mice, neurobehavioural development in rats and perinatal survival in mink, fall within a very small range (Table 9). Based on the lowest reported NOELs included in the table (approximately 0.05 mg/kg body weight per day based primarily on hepatic effects observed in a subchronic study in pigs and in chronic studies in rats), a TDI of 0.17 µg/kg body weight per day has been derived for non-neoplastic effects, by incorporating an uncertainty factor of 300 (x 10 for intraspecies variation; x 10 for interspecies variation, x 3 for severity of effect). A factor of 3 for severity of effects was chosen as HCB causes i) multiple non-neoplastic effects in several species, and ii) LOELs for a number of end-points for which NOELs have not been determined are very close to the NOEL, from the critical studies, of 0.05 mg/kg body weight per day. However, it is fully realized that national authorities may choose other end-points or uncertainty factors depending upon data evaluation and future scientific findings.

10.1.3.2 Neoplastic effects

The approach for neoplastic effects is based on the Tumorigenic Dose$_5$, or TD_5 i.e., the intake or exposure associated with a 5% excess incidence of tumours in experimental studies in animals (IPCS, 1994). This is a benchmark approach in which the TD_5 is calculated directly from the experimental data rather than using the upper or lower confidence limits. Uncertainty factors are then applied to the TD_5 to obtain a guidance value. The choice of uncertainty factors is based on the level and nature of mechanistic data available, the quality of the database, the tumour pattern, the dose-response relationship, and the experimental model chosen. The final value will reflect the degree of certainty one has with the available information.

For the purpose of indicating the magnitude of risk of HCB, the two-generation study in rats has been selected, owing to its relevance to the exposure of the general human population, as the design of this study involved exposure to relatively low concentrations of HCB in the diet (including *in utero* and lactational exposure). Moreover, tumour pathology was inadequately reported in the available studies in hamsters and mice, and there is some concern that in the other adequate study in rats, there may also have been exposure by inhalation to some HCB that was incorporated in the diet as a powder.

The TD_5 value was calculated from the results of the two-generation study in rats using a multistage model (Crump & Howe, 1982). The tumour incidences in the pups were analysed in the same manner as data from a single-generation study, owing to the lack of information on individual litters. On this basis, the TD_5 values range from 0.81 mg/kg body weight per day for neoplastic liver nodules in females to 2.01 mg/kg body weight per day for parathyroid adenomas in males. The Task Group decided that the most sensitive end-point (neoplastic nodules of the liver) would be used in its analysis. In calculating the suggested guidance value, it was agreed to use an uncertainty factor of 5000, based on consideration of the insufficient mechanistic data. The TD_5 was divided by this uncertainty factor to arrive at the suggested guidance value of 0.16 µg/kg body weight per day. However, it is fully realized that national authorities may choose other end-points or uncertainty factors depending upon data evaluation and future scientific findings.

Although infants may have a high intake of HCB via breast milk for a short time, the TD_5 and TDI were considered to be protective of the health of this population (unless there are extreme exposures), because one of the long-term studies used in deriving these values included lactational exposure. However, it should be noted that the TD_5 and TDI values derived above should not be compared directly with intakes from breast milk by nursing infants, since the guidance values are based on a lifetime intake, whereas the duration of breast-feeding is relatively short.

10.2 Evaluation of effects on the environment

HCB is widely distributed in the environment, by virtue of its mobility and resistance to degradation, although slow photodegradation in air (half-life of approximately 80 days) and microbial degradation (half-life of several years) do occur. It has been detected in air, water, sediment, soil and biota from around the world. HCB is a bioaccumulative substance (BCF values range from 375 to > 35 000), and biomagnification of HCB through the food chain has been reported.

In studies of the acute toxicity of HCB to aquatic organisms, exposure to concentrations in the range of 1 to 17 µg/litre reduced production of chlorophyll in algae and reproduction in ciliate protozoa. In longer-term studies, the growth of sensitive freshwater algae and protozoa was affected by a concentration of 1 µg/litre, while a concentration of approximately 3 µg/litre caused mortality in amphipods and liver necrosis in largemouth bass. The concentrations of HCB in surface waters around the world are much lower than these effect levels (3 to 5 orders of magnitude lower), except in a few extremely contaminated localities.

Injection studies in eggs have shown that tissue levels of 1500 ng/g wet weight reduce embryo weights in herring gulls (lowest dose tested). No studies were available to establish a NOAEL. For many bird species, reduced embryo weights are associated with lower survival of chicks. This effect level is within an order of magnitude of the levels measured in the eggs of sea birds and raptors from a number of locations from around the world, suggesting that present levels of HCB in certain locations may harm embryos of bird species.

Experimental studies on mink indicate that they are sensitive to the toxic effects of HCB; long-term ingestion of diets containing 1000 ng HCB/g (the lowest dose tested) increased mortality, decreased birth weights of offspring exposed *in utero* and via lactation, and altered levels of neurotransmitters in the hypothalamus of dams and their offspring. No studies were available to establish a NOAEL. This dietary effect level is only a few times higher than the concentrations of HCB measured in various species of fish from a number of industrialized locations from around the world, suggesting that present levels of HCB in fish species from certain locations may adversely affect mink and perhaps other fish-eating mammals.

11. RECOMMENDATION FOR PROTECTION OF HUMAN HEALTH AND THE ENVIRONMENT

a) Alternatives should be found for any present uses of HCB.

b) It is important to reduce the environmental burden of HCB by: (i) identifying remaining sources and quantities of release to the environment from these sources, including point source emissions, waste disposal sites and production facilities; (ii) applying appropriate manufacturing and waste disposal practices in order to decrease levels of HCB in the environment.

c) Human monitoring of HCB in blood and breast milk should be undertaken to develop data representing exposure of the general population, in order to identify highly exposed populations and potential sources, and to enable interpretation of individual results.

d) In order to gauge the efficacy of control measures it would be valuable to monitor environmental levels and effects in locations where levels are higher than the global average.

e) Neonatal effects in humans and other species have been associated with ingestion of high doses of HCB through breast milk. It is recommended that techniques be developed to assess appropriately the risk to infant health from exposure to HCB and related compounds in breast milk.

12. FURTHER RESEARCH

12.1 Environment

a) To improve the database available for environmental risk assessment, it is considered important to establish a NOEL for the serious reproductive effects seen in mink at dietary levels approaching those found in certain locations.

b) Since HCB is persistent in soil and sediment, it would be valuable to perform biodiversity experiments with HCB-treated soil and sediment.

12.2 Human health

a) Based on the effects of low doses of HCB on ovarian tissues in primates, involving disorders of germ cells and the ovarian surface epithelium, the following is recommended:

  (i) exposed populations should be studied for relevant reproductive human outcomes of interest, particularly, fetal loss and ovarian cancer;

  (ii) reproductive tissues such as ovarian follicular fluid should be included in human monitoring studies on HCB levels and/or effects.

b) In order to decrease uncertainty in the risk assessment of HCB and related compounds, research into the primary mechanism(s) of action for tumorigenic, thyroid, reproductive, porphyrigenic, neurotoxic and immunological effects of HCB should be undertaken.

c) Preliminary evidence suggests that HCB acts, at least in part, through Ah receptor-linked mechanisms. This should be evaluated more fully and compared to other polyhalogenated aromatic chemicals for which a wealth of data are already available.

d) Given the toxicity of HCB and the few data for humans, multicentre longitudinal studies of highly exposed human populations should be undertaken. End-points of interest should cover toxicokinetics (e.g., half-life), thyroid function, porphyrin metabolism, reproductive outcomes (e.g., fetal losses), and cancer. Nursing infants from these populations should be followed to assess immunological and neurobehavioural development.

13. PREVIOUS EVALUATIONS BY INTERNATIONAL BODIES

The International Agency for Research on Cancer has classified HCB as a Group 2B carcinogen (possibly carcinogenic to humans) based on inadequate evidence for carcinogenicity to humans and sufficient evidence for carcinogenicity to animals (IARC, 1987).

A drinking-water guideline of 1 μg/litre was developed for HCB based on an evaluation of the production of liver tumours in female rats and applying the linearized multistage model to calculate an excess life-time cancer risk of 10^{-5} (WHO, 1993).

A conditional acceptable daily intake of 0.6 μg HCB/kg body weight was developed by the Joint FAO/WHO Joint Meeting on Pesticide Residues in Food (FAO/WHO, 1975). This recommendation was withdrawn in 1978 (FAO/WHO, 1978).

Regulatory standards established by national bodies in different countries and the European Union are summarized in the Legal File of the International Register of Potentially Toxic Chemicals (IRPTC, 1993).

REFERENCES

Abbott DC, Collins GB, & Goulding R (1972) Organochlorine pesticide residues in human fat in the United Kingdom 1969-71. Br Med J, **2**: 533-556.

Abbott DC, Collins GB, Goulding R, & Hoodless RA (1981) Organochlorine pesticide residues in human fat in the United Kingdom 1976-77. Br Med J, **283**: 1425-1428.

Abbott DC, Goulding R, Holmes DC, & Hoodless RA (1985) Organochlorine pesticide residues in human fat in the United Kingdom 1982-1983. Hum Toxicol, **4**: 435-445.

Abraham K, Hille A, Ende M, & Helge H (1994) Intake and fecal excretion of PCDDs, PCDFs, HCB and PCBs (138, 153, 180) in a breast-fed and a formula-fed infant. Chemosphere, **29**(9-11): 2279-2286.

Ahling B, Bjorseth A, & Lunde G (1978) Formation of chlorinated hydrocarbons during combustion of poly(vinyl chloride). Chemosphere, **10**: 799-806.

Ahmad N, Benoit D, Brooke L, Call D, Carlson A, Defoe D, Huot J, Moriarity A, Richter J, Shubat P, Veith G, & Wallbridge C (1984) Aquatic toxicity tests to characterize the hazard of volatile organic chemicals in water: A toxicity data summary, Parts I and II. Duluth, Minnesota, US Environmental Protection Agency, Environmental Research Laboratory (EPA 600/3-84-009).

Albert LA, Alpuche L, Barcenas C, & Rendón J (1990) A survey of organochlorine pesticide residues in cheese samples from three Mexican regions. Environ Pollut, **65**: 119-126.

Albro PW & Thomas R(1974) Intestinal absorption of hexachlorobenzene and hexachlorocyclohexane isomers in rats. Bull Environ Contam Toxicol, **12**: 289-294.

Alves HHD & Chevalier M (1980) L'hexachlorobenzène dans l'environnement québécois : Production, utilisation et présence. Montréal, Québec, Environnement Canada, Service de la Protection de l'Environnement (Rapport No EPS-3 QR-80-1).

Andrews JE & Courtney KD (1986) Hexachlorobenzene-induced renal maldevelopment in CD-1 mice and CD rats. In: Morris CR & Cabral JRP ed. Hexachlorobenzene: Proceedings of an International Symposium. Lyon, International Agency for Research on Cancer, pp 381-391 (IARC Scientific Publications No. 77).

Andrews JE, Courtney KD, Stead AG, & Donaldson WE (1989) Hexachlorobenzene induced hyperparathyroidism and osteosclerosis in rats. Fundam Appl Toxicol, **12**: 242-251.

Andrews JE, Jackson LD, Stead AG, & Donaldson WE (1990) Morphometric analysis of osteosclerotic bone resulting from hexachlorobenzene exposure. J Toxicol Environ Health, **31**: 193-201.

Angerer J, Heinzow B, Reimann DO, Knorz W, & Lehnert G (1992) Internal exposure to organic substances in a municipal waste incinerator. Int Arch Occup Environ Health, **64**: 265-273.

Ariño AA, Herrera A, Conchello MP, & Pérez C (1992) Hexachlorobenzene residues in Spanish meat products after cooking, curing, and long-term ripening. J Food Prot, **55**(11): 920-923.

Ariño A, Herrera A, Conchello P, & Lazaro R (1993) Hexachlorobenzene and hexachlorocyclohexane residues in pork as affected by weight and sex. Bull Environ Contam Toxicol, **51**: 647-650.

Arnold DL & Krewski D (1988) Long-term toxicity of hexachlorobenzene. Food Chem Toxicol, **26**: 169-174.

Arnold DL, Moodie CA, Charbonneau SM, Grice HC, McGuire PF, Bryce FR, Collins BT, Zwadizka ZZ, Krewski DR, Nera EA, & Munro IC (1985) Long-term toxicity of hexachlorobenzene in the rat and the effect of dietary vitamin A. Food Chem Toxicol, **23**: 779-793.

Atlas E & Giam CS (1981) Global transport of organic pollutants: ambient concentrations in the remote marine atmosphere. Science, **211**: 163-165.

ATSDR (1990) Toxicological profile for hexachlorobenzene. Atlanta, Georgia, Agency for Toxic Substances and Disease Registry (TP-90-17).

ATSDR (1994) Toxicological profile for hexachlorobenzene - Update. Atlanta, Georgia, Agency for Toxic Substances and Disease Registry.

Atuma SS, Andersson O, Linder C-E, & Hansson L (1993) Levels of some organochlorine compounds in sea trout (*Salmo trutta*) and whitefish (*Caregonus lavaretus*) from the Gulf of Bothnia. Aqua Fenn, **23**: 221-226.

Avrahami M (1975) Hexachlorobenzene: IV. Accumulation and elimination of HCB by pigs after oral dosing. NZ J Exp Agric, **3**: 285-287.

Avrahami M & Steele RT (1972) Hexachlorobenzene: I. Accumulation and elimination of HCB in sheep after oral dosing. NZ J Agric Res, **15**: 476-481.

Ayotte P, Dewailly E, Bruneau S, Careau H, & Vézina A (1995) Arctic air pollution and human health: what effects should be expected? Sci Total Environ, **160/161**: 529-537.

Babineau KA, Singh A, Jarrell JF, & Villeneuve DC (1991) Surface epithelium of the ovary following oral administration of hexachlorobenzene to the monkey. J Submicrosc Cytol Pathol, **23**: 457-464.

Bailey J, Knauf V, Mueller W, & Hobson W (1980) Transfer of hexachlorobenzene and polychlorinated biphenyls to nursing infant rhesus monkeys; enhanced toxicity. Environ Res, **21**: 190-196.

Ballschmiter K, & Wittlinger R (1991) Interhemisphere exchange of hexachlorocyclohexanes, hexachlorobenzene, polychlorobiphenyls, and 1,1,1-trichloro-2,2-bis-(p-chlorophenyl)ethane in the lower troposphere. Environ Sci Technol, **25**: 1103-1111.

Barnett JB, Barfield L, Walls R, Joyner R, Owens R, & Soderberg LSF (1987) The effect of in utero exposure to hexachlorobenzene on the developing immune response of BALB/c mice. Toxicol Lett, **39**: 263-274.

Barquet A, Morgade C, & Pfaffenberger CD (1981) Determination of organochlorine pesticides and metabolites in drinking water, human blood serum, and adipose tissue. J Toxicol Environ Health, **7**: 469-479.

Bates MN, Hannah DJ, Buckland SJ, Taucher JA, & Van Maanen T (1994) Chlorinated organic contaminants in breast milk of New Zealand women. Environ Health Perspect, **102** (Suppl 1): 211-217.

Bauer I, Weigelt S, & Ernst W (1989) Biotransformation of hexachlorobenzene in the blue mussel (*Mytilus edulis*). Chemosphere, **19**(10/11): 1701-1707.

Beck J & Hansen KE (1974) The degradation of quintozene, pentachlorobenzene, hexachlorobenzene and pentachloroaniline in soil. Pestic Sci, **5**: 41-48.

Béland P, Deguise S, & Plante R (1991) Toxicology and pathology of St. Lawrence marine mammals - Final report. Rimouski, Québec, Canada, Wildlife Toxicology Fund Research Grant, St. Lawrence National Institute of Ecotoxicology, 95 pp.

Belfroid A, Van Wezel A, Sikkenk M, Van Gestel K, Seinen W, & Hermens J (1993) The toxicokinetic behaviour of chlorobenzenes in earthworms (*Eisenia andrei*): Experiments in water. Ecotoxicol Environ Saf, **25**: 154-165.

Belfroid A, Meiling J, Sijm D, Hermens J, Seinen W, & Van Gestel K (1994a) Uptake of hydrophobic halogenated aromatic hydrocarbons from food by earthworms (*Eisenia andrei*). Arch Environ Contam Toxicol, **27**: 260-265.

Belfroid A, Sikkenk M, Seinen W, Van Gestel K, & Hermens J (1994b) The toxicokinetic behavior of chlorobenzenes in earthworm (*Eisenia andrei*): Experiments in soil. Environ Toxicol Chem, **13**: 93-99.

Beretta M & Dick T (1994) Organochlorine compounds in human milk, Porto Alegre, Brazil. Bull Environ Contam Toxicol, **53**: 357-360.

Biddleman TF, Billings WN, & Foreman WT (1986) Vapor-particle partitioning of semivolatile organic compounds: Estimates from field collection. Environ Sci Technol, **20**: 1038-1043.

Bidleman TF, Wideqvist U, Jansson B, & Soderlund R (1987) Organochlorine pesticides and polychlorinated biphenyls in the atmosphere of southern Sweden. Atmos Environ, **21**: 641-654.

Bidleman TF, Walla MD, Roura R, Carr E, & Schmidt S (1993) Organochlorine pesticides in the atmosphere of the Southern Ocean and Antarctica, January-March, 1990. Mar Pollut Bull, **26**(5): 258-262.

Billings WN & Bidleman TF (1980) Field comparison of polyurethane foam and Teax-GC resin for high-volume air sampling of chlorinated hydrocarbons. Environ Sci Technol, **14**(6):679-683.

Bishop CA, Lean DRS, Brooks RJ, Carey JH, & Ng P (1995) Chlorinated hydrocarbons in early life stages of the common snapping turtle (*Chelydra serpentina serpentina*) from a coastal wetland on Lake Ontario, Canada. Environ Toxicol Chem, **14**(3): 421-426.

Bjerk JE & Brevik EM (1980) Organochlorine compounds in aquatic environments. Arch Environ Contam Toxicol, **9**: 743-750.

Bleavins MR, Breslin WJ, Aulerich RJ, & Ringer RK (1982) Excretion and placental and mammary transfer of hexachlorobenzene in the European ferret (*Mustela putorius furo*). J Toxicol Environ Health, **14**: 929-940.

Bleavins MR, Bursian SJ, Brewster JS, & Aulerich RJ (1984a) Effects of dietary hexachlorobenzene exposure on regional brain biogenic amine concentrations in mink and European ferrets. J Toxicol Environ Health, **14**: 363-377.

Bleavins MR, Aulerich RJ, & Ringer RK (1984b) Effects of chronic dietary hexachlorobenzene exposure on the reproductive performance and survivability of mink and European ferrets. Arch Environ Contam Toxicol, **13**: 357-365.

Boersma DC, Ellenton JL, & Yagminas A (1986) Investigation of the hepatic mixed-function oxidase system in herring gull embryos in relation to environmental contaminants. Environ Toxicol Chem, **5**: 309-318.

Boese BL, Winsor M, Lee H II, Specht DT, & Rukavina LC (1990) Depuration kinetics of hexachlorobenzene in the clam, *Macoma nasuta*. Comp Biochem Physiol, **C996**: 327-331.

Bordet F, Mallet J, Maurice L, Borrel S, & Venant A (1993) Organochlorine pesticide and PCB congener content of French human milk. Bull Environ Contam Toxicol, **50**: 425-432.

Bourbonniere RA, Van Sickle BL, & Mayer T (1986) The Great Lakes sediment bank-I (including catalogs of lakes Huron and Ontario samples). Burlington, Ontario, Environment Canada, National Water Research Institute (NWRI Contribution No. 86-151).

Bouthillier L, Greselin E, Brodeur J, Viau C, & Charbonneau M (1991) Male rat specific nephrotoxicity resulting from subchronic administration of hexachlorobenzene. Toxicol Appl Pharmacol, **110**: 315-326.

Braune BM & Norstrom RJ (1989) Dynamics of organochlorine compounds in herring gulls: III. Tissue distribution and bioaccumulation in Lake Ontario gulls. Environ Toxicol Chem, **8**: 957-968.

Breslin WJ, Bleavins MR, & Ringer RK (1983) Distribution and excretion of hexachlorobenzene in bobwhite. J Toxicol Environ Health, **11:** 885-896.

Brooks GW & Hunt GE (1984) Source assessment for hexachlorobenzene. Research Triangle Park, North Carolina, Radian Corporation (Prepared for the US Environmental Protection Agency, Research Triangle Park) (EPA 68-02-3818).

Bro-Rasmussen F (1986) Hexachlorobenzene: An ecotoxicological profile of an organochlorine compound. In: Morris CR & Cabral JRP ed. Hexachlorobenzene: Proceedings of an International Symposium. Lyon, International Agency for Research on Cancer, pp 231-239 (IARC Scientific Publications No. 77).

Brown EA, Biddle K, & Spaulding JE (1986) Residue levels of hexachlorobenzene in meat and poultry in the food supply of the U.S.A. In: Morris CR & Cabral JRPed. Hexachlorobenzene: Proceedings of an International Symposium. Lyon, International Agency for Research on Cancer, pp 99-108 (IARC Scientific Publications No. 77).

Bruckmann P, Kersten W, Funcke W, Balfanz E, Konig J, Theisen J, Ball M, & Papke O (1988) The occurrence of chlorinated and other organic trace compounds in urban air. Chemosphere, **17**: 2363-1380.

Brunn H & Manz D (1982) Contamination of native fish stock by hexachlorobenzene and polychlorinated biphenyl residues. Bull Environ Contam Toxicol, **28**: 599-604.

Brusick DJ (1986) Genotoxicity of hexachlorobenzene and other chlorinated benzenes. In: Morris CR & Cabral JRP ed. Hexachlorobenzene: Proceedings of an International Symposium. Lyon, International Agency for Research on Cancer, pp 393-397 (IARC Scientific Publications No. 77).

BUA (German Chemical Society-Advisory Committee on Existing Chemicals of Environmental Relevance) (1994) Hexachlorobenzene. Stuttgart, S. Hirzel Wissenschaftliche Verlagsgesellschaft, 257 pp (BUA Report 119).

Buhler DR & Carpenter HM (1986) Japanese quail as a model for the study of hexachlorobenzene-induced porphyria. In: Morris CR & Cabral JRP ed. Hexachlorobenzene:

Proceedings of an International Symposium. Lyon, International Agency for Research on Cancer, pp 477-480 (IARC Scientific Publications No. 77).

Burns JE & Miller FM (1975) Hexachlorobenzene contamination: its effects in a Louisiana population. Arch Environ Health, **30**: 44-48.

Burns JE, Miller FM, Gomes ED, & Albert RA (1974) Hexachlorobenzene exposure from contaminated DCPA in vegetable spraymen. Arch Environ Health, **29**: 192-194.

Burton MA & Bennett BG (1987) Exposure of man to environmental hexachlorobenzene (HCB): an exposure commitment assessment. Sci Total Environ, **66**: 137-146.

Bush B, Snow J, Connor S, & Koblintz R (1985) Polychlorinated biphenyl congeners (PCBs), p,p′-DDe and hexachlorobenzene in human milk in three areas of upstate New York. Arch Environ Contam Toxicol, **14**: 443-450.

Cabral JRP & Shubik P (1986) Carcinogenic activity of hexachlorobenzene in mice and hamsters. In: Morris CR & Cabral JRP ed. Hexachlorobenzene: Proceedings of an International Symposium. Lyon, International Agency for Research on Cancer, pp 411-416 (IARC Scientific Publications No. 77).

Cabral JRP, Shubik P, Mollner T, & Raitano F (1977) Carcinogenic activity of hexachlorobenzene in hamsters. Nature (Lond), **269**: 510-511.

Cabral JRP, Mollner T, Raitano F, & Shubik P (1979) Carcinogenesis of hexachlorobenzene in mice. Int J Cancer, **23**: 47-51.

Calamari D, Galassi S, Setti F, & Vighi M (1983) Toxicity of selected chlorobenzenes to aquatic organisms. Chemosphere, **12**: 253-262.

Call DJ, Brooke LT, Ahmad N, & Richter JE (1983) Toxicity and metabolism studies with EPA priority pollutants and related chemicals in freshwater organisms. Center for Lake Superior Environmental Studies, University of Wisconsin-Superior, Environmental Research Laboratory, Duluth, Minnesota, U.S. Environmental Protection Agency (EPA 600/3-83-095).

Callahan M, Slimak M, Gabel N, May I, Fowler C, Freed R, Jennings P, Durfee R, Whitmore F, Maestri B, Mabey W, Holt B, & Gould C (1979) Water-related environmental fate of 129 priority pollutants, Volume II. Washington, DC, US Environmental Protection Agency, Office of Water Planning and Standards/Office of Water and Waste Management (EPA 440/4-79-029b).

Cam C (1960) Une nouvelle dermatose épidémique des enfants. Ann Dermatol, **87**: 393-397.

Cam C & Nigogosyan G (1963) Acquired toxic porphyria cutanea tarda due to hexachlorobenzene. J Am Med Assoc, **183**: 90-93.

Camps M, Planas J, Gómez-Catalán J, Sabroso M, To-Figueras J, & Corbella J (1989) Organochlorine residues in human adipose tissue in Spain: study of an agrarian area. Bull Environ Contam Toxicol, **42**: 195-201.

Carey AE, Gowen JA, Tai H, Mitchell WG, & Wiersma GB (1979) Pesticide residue levels in soils and crops from 37 states, 1972 - National Soils Monitoring Program (IV). Pest. Monit. J, **12**: 209-229.

Carey AE, Dixon TE, & Yang HSC (1985) Environmental exposure to hexachlorobenzene in the United States. Washington, DC, US Environmental Protection Agency, Office of Pesticides and Toxic Substances.

Carlson AR & Kosian PA (1987) Toxicity of chlorinated benzenes to fathead minnows (*Pimephales promelas*). Arch Environ Contam Toxicol, **16**: 129-135.

Carthew P & Smith AG (1994) Pathological mechanisms of hepatic tumour formation in rats exposed chronically to dietary hexachlorobenzene. J Appl Toxicol, **14**: 447-452.

Carthew P, Edwards RE, & Smith AG (1990) Immunotoxic effects of hexachlorobenzene on the pathogenesis of systemic, pneumonic and hepatic virus infections in the mouse. Hum Exp Toxicol, **8**: 403-411.

Clark TP, Norstrom RJ, Fox GA, & Won HT (1987) Dynamics of organochlorine compounds in herring gulls (*Larus argentatus*): II. A two-compartment model and data for ten compounds. Environ Toxicol Chem, **6:** 547-559.

Conchello P, Herrera A, Ariño A, Lazaro R, & Pérez-Arquillué C (1993) Effect of grilling, roasting, and cooking on the natural hexachlorobenzene content of ovine meat. Bull Environ Contam Toxicol, **50**: 828-833.

Conde C, Naluenda C, & Arrabal C (1993) Hexachlorobenzene (HCB) in human milk in Spain from 1984 to 1991. Bull Environ Contam Toxicol, **51**: 827-831.

Courtney KD (1979) Hexachlorobenzene (HCB): a review. Environ Res, **20**: 225-266.

Courtney KD & Andrews JE (1979) Mobilization of hexachlorobenzene (HCB) during gestation. Toxicol Lett, **3**: 357-361.

Courtney KD & Andrews JE (1985) Neonatal and maternal body burdens of hexachlorobenzene (HCB) in mice: gestational exposure and lactational transfer. Fundam Appl Toxicol, **5**: 265-277.

Courtney KD, Copeland MF, & Robbins A (1976) The effects of pentachloronitrobenzene, hexachlorobenzene, and related compounds on fetal development. Toxicol Appl Pharmacol, **35**: 239-256.

Courtney KD, Andrews JE, & Svendsgaard DJ (1979) Hexachlorobenzene (HCB) deposition in maternal and fetal tissues of rat and mouse: I. Chemical quantification of HCB in tissues. Environ Res, **19**: 1-13.

Cripps DJ, Peters HA, Gocmen A, & Dogramaci I (1984) Porphyria turcica due to hexachlorobenzene: a 20 to 30 year follow-up study on 204 patients. Br J Dermatol, **111**: 413-422.

Cross JN, Hardy JT, Hose JE, Hershelman GP, Antrim LD, Gossett RW, & Crecelius EA (1987) Contaminant concentrations and toxicity of sea-surface microlayer near Los Angeles, California. Mar Environ Res, **23**: 307-323.

Crump K & Howe N (1982) Global '82: a computer program to extrapolate quantal animal toxicity data to low doses (Contract #41USC252C3). Washington, DC, US Occupational Safety and Health Administration, Office of Carcinogen Standards.

Currier MF, McClimans CD, & Barna-Lloyd G (1980) Hexachlorobenzene blood levels and the health status of men employed in the manufacture of chlorinated solvents. J Toxicol Environ Health, **6**: 367-377.

D'Amour M & Charbonneau M (1992) Sex-related differences in hepatic glutathione conjugation of hexachlorobenzene in the rat. Toxicol Appl Pharmacol, **112**: 229-234.

Davies K (1988) Concentrations and dietary intake of selected organochlorines, including PCBs, PCDDs and PCDFs in fresh food composites grown in Ontario, Canada. Chemosphere, **17**: 263-276.

Davis BD & Morgan RC (1986) Hexachlorobenzene in hazardous waste sites. In: Morris CR & Cabral JRP ed. Hexachlorobenzene: Proceedings of an International Symposium. Lyon, International Agency for Research on Cancer, pp 23-30 (IARC Scientific Publications No. 77).

Debets FMH & Strik JJTWA (1979) An approach to elucidate the mechanism of hexachlorobenzene-induced hepatic porphyria, as a model for the hepatotoxicity of polyhalogenated aromatic compounds (PHA's). In: Strik JJTWA & Koeman JH ed. Chemical porphyria in man. Amsterdam, Oxford, New York, Elsevier/North Holland Biomedical Press, pp 181-208.

Deleon IR, Maberry MA, Overton EB, Raschke CK, Remele PC, Steele, CF, Warren VL, & Laseter JL (1980) Rapid gas chromatographic method for the determination of volatile and semivolatile organochlorine compounds in soil and chemical waste disposal site samples. J Chromatogr Sci, **18**: 85-88.

Dellinger B, Taylor PH, & Tirey DA (1991) Minimization and control of hazardous combustion by-products. Cincinnati, Ohio, US Environmental Protection Agency, Risk Reduction Laboratory (EPA 600/S2-90/039).

De Matteis F, Prior BE, & Rimington C (1961) Nervous and biochemical disturbances following hexachlorobenzene intoxication. Nature (Lond), **191**(4786): 363-366.

Den Besten C, Bennik MM, Van Iersel M, Peters MA, Teunis C, & Van Bladeren PJ (1994) Comparison of the urinary metabolite profiles of hexachlorobenzene and pentachlorobenzene in the rat. Chem-Biol Interact, **90**: 121-137.

Den Desten C, Bennik MHJ, Bruggeman I, Schielen P, Kuper F, Brouwer A, Koeman JH, Vos JG, & Van Bladeren PJ (1993) The role of oxidative metabolism in hexachlorobenzene-induced porphyria and thyroid hormone homeostasis: a comparison with pentachlorobenzene in a 13-week feeding study. Toxicol Appl Pharmacol, **119**: 181-194.

Denomme MA, Leece B, Gyorkos J, Homonko K, & Safe S (1983) Polychlorinated benzene and phenol congeners as inducers of rat hepatic drug-metabolizing enzymes in immature male Wistar rats. Can J Physiol Pharmacol, **61**: 1063-1070.

Den Tonkelaar EM & Van Esch GJ (1974) No-effect levels of organochlorine pesticides based on induction of microsomal liver enzymes in short-term toxicity experiments. Toxicology, **2**: 371-380.

Den Tonkelaar EM, Verschueren HG, Bankovska J, De Vries T, Kroes R, & Van Esch G (1978) Hexachlorobenzene toxicity in pigs. Toxicol Appl Pharmacol, **43**: 137-145.

Devault DS (1985) Contaminants in fish from Great Lakes harbors and tributary mouths. Arch Environ Contam Toxicol, **14**: 587-594.

Dewailly E, Nantel A, Laliberté C, Weber J-P, Gingras S, & Meyer F (1991) Organochlorines in the breast milk in Québec: a provincial survey. Poster presentation at the Conference on Measuring, Understanding, and Predicting Exposures in the 21st Century, Atlanta, Georgia, 18-22 November 1991.

Ding W-H, Aldous KM, Briggs RG, Valente H, Hilker DR, Connor S, & Eadon GA (1992) Application of multivariate statistical analysis to evaluate local sources of chlorobenzene congeners in soil samples. Chemosphere, **25**(5): 675-690.

Dogramaci I (1964) Porphyrias and porphyrin metabolism with special reference to porphyria in childhood. Adv Pediatr, **13**: 11-63.

Dogramaci I, Wray JD, Ergene T, Sezer V, & Müftü Y (1962) Porphyria turcica: a survey of 592 cases of cutaneous porphyria seen in southeastern Turkey. Turk J Pediatr, **4**: 138-148.

Eisenberg M & Topping JJ (1984) Organochlorine residues in shellfish from Maryland waters. J Environ Sci Health, **B19**: 673-688.

Eisenreich SJ & Strachan WMJ (1992) Estimating atmospheric deposition of toxic substances to the Great Lakes - An update: Proceedings of a workshop, Burlington, 31 January-2 February 1992. Burlington, Ontario, Canada Centre for Inland Waters.

El-Dib MA & Badawy MI (1985) Organochlorine insecticides and PCBs in waste, sediment, and fish from the Mediterranean Sea. Bull Environ Contam Toxicol, **34**: 216-227.

Elissalde MH & Clark DE (1979) Testosterone metabolism by hexachlorobenzene-induced hepatic microsomal enzymes. Am J Vet Res, **40**: 1762-1766.

Elkin BT & Bethke RW (1995) Environmental contaminants in caribou in the Northwest Territories, Canada. Sci Total Environ, **160/161**: 307-321.

Enriquez De Salamanca R, Lopez-Miras A, Munoz JJ, To-Figueras J, & Conde C (1990) Is hexachlorobenzene human overload related to porphyria cutanea tarda? A speculative hypothesis. Med Hypotheses, **33**: 69-71.

Environment Canada (1989) Atlantic region federal-provincial toxic chemical survey of municipal drinking water sources 1985-1988 - Interpretative Report. Moncton, New Brunswick, Environment Canada, Conservation and Protection, Water Quality Branch, Inland Waters Directorate.

Environment Canada (1992) Detroit incinerator monitoring program: Data report No. 6. Ottawa, Ontario, Environment Canada, Conservation and Protection, River Road Environmental Technology Centre (Report No. PMD-92-1).

Environment Canada/Department of Fisheries & Oceans/Health & Welfare Canada (1991) Toxic chemicals in the Great Lakes and associated effects - Volume 1: Contaminant levels and trends. Ottawa, Ontario, Minister of Supply and Services.

Environment Canada/Ontario Ministry of the Environment (1986) St. Clair River pollution investigation (Sarnia area). Toronto, Canada-Ontario Agreement Respecting Great Lakes Water Quality.

Ernst W (1986) Hexachlorobenzene in the marine environment: distribution, fate and ecotoxicological aspects. In: Morris CR & Cabral JRP ed. Hexachlorobenzene: Proceedings of an International Symposium. Lyon, International Agency for Research on Cancer, pp 211-222 (IARC Scientific Publications No. 77).

Erturk E, Lambrecht RW, Grunden EE, Headley DB, Peters HA, Morris CR, & Bryan GT (1982) Leukemogenicity of hexachlorobenzene (HCB) in Swiss mice (SM) after subchronic feeding. Proc Am Assoc Cancer Res, **23**: 55 (Abstract).

Ertürk E, Lambrecht RW, Peters HA, Cripps DJ, Gocmen A, Morris CR, & Bryan GT (1986) Oncogenicity of hexachlorobenzene. In: Morris CR & Cabral JRP ed. Hexachlorobenzene: Proceedings of an International Symposium. Lyon, International Agency for Research on Cancer, pp 417-423 (IARC Scientific Publications No. 77).

Falandysz J & Szefer P (1982) Chlorinated hydrocarbons in diving ducks wintering in Gdansk Bay, Baltic Sea. Sci Total Environ, **24:** 119-127.

Falandysz J, Kannan K, Tanabe S, & Tatukawa R (1993) Persistent organochlorine residues in canned cod-livers of the southern Baltic origin. Bull Environ Contam Toxicol, **50:** 929-934.

FAO/WHO (1975) Report of the Joint Meeting of FAO Working Party of Experts on Pesticide Residues and the WHO Expert Committee on Pesticide Residues. Geneva, World Health Organization, 37 pp (WHO Technical Report Series 574).

FAO/WHO (1978) Pesticide residues in food - 1978. Report of the Joint Meeting of the FAO Panel of Experts on Pesticide Residues and Environment and the WHO Expert Group on Pesticide Residues. Rome, Food and Agriculture Organization of the United Nations, pp 19-20 (FAO Plant Production and Protection Paper 15).

Ferrer A, Bona MA, Castellano M, To-Figueras J, & Brunet M (1992) Organochlorine residues in human adipose tissue of the population of Zaragoza (Spain). Bull Environ Contam Toxicol, **48**: 561-566.

Fingler S, Drevenkar V, Tkalčević B, & Šmit Z (1992) Levels of polychlorinated biphenyls, organochlorine pesticides, and chlorophenols in the Kupa River water and in drinking waters from different areas in Croatia. Bull Environ Contam Toxicol, **49**: 805-812.

Foley RE & Batcheller GR (1988) Organochlorine contaminants in common goldeneye wintering on the Niagara River. J Wildl Manage, **52:** 441-445.

Foster WG, McMahon A, Jarrell JF, & Villeneuve DC (1992a) Hexachlorobenzene (HCB) suppresses circulating progesterone concentrations during the luteal phase in the cynomolgus monkey. J Appl Toxicol, **12**: 13-17.

Foster WG, Pentick JA, McMahon A, & Lecavalier PR (1992b) Ovarian toxicity of hexachlorobenzene (HCB) in the superovulated female rat. J Biochem Toxicol, **7**: 1-4.

Foster WG, Pentick JA, McMahon A, & Lecavalier PR (1993) Body distribution and endocrine toxicity of hexachlorobenzene (HCB) in the female rat. J Appl Toxicol, **13**: 79-83.

Foster WG, Mertineit C, Yagminas A, McMahon A, & Lecavalier P (1995) The effects of hexachlorobenzene on circulating levels of adrenal steroids in the ovariectomized rat. J Biochem Toxicol, **10**(3): 129-135.

Fox ME, Carey JH, & Olivier BG (1983) Compartmental distribution of organochlorine contaminants in the Niagara River and the Western Basin of Lake Ontario. J Great Lakes Res, **9**: 287-294.

Franchi E & Focardi S (1991) Polychlorinated biphenyl congeners, hexachlorobenzene and DDT in human milk in central Italy. Sci Total Environ, **102**: 223-228.

Frank R & Ripley BD (1990) Food residues from pesticides and environmental pollutants in Ontario. In: Nriagu JO & Simmons MS ed. Food contamination from environmental sources. New York, Wiley-Interscience, pp 473-524.

Frank R, Braun HE, & Fleming G (1983) Organochlorine and organophosphorus residues in fat of bovine and porcine carcasses marketed in Ontario, Canada from 1969 to 1981. J Food Prot, **46**: 893-900.

Frank R, Braun HE, Sirons GH, Rasper J, & Ward GG (1985a) Organochlorine and organophosphorus insecticides and industrial pollutants in the milk supplies of Ontario - 1983. J Food Prot, **48**: 499-504.

Frank R, Rasper J, Braun HE, & Ashton G (1985b) Disappearance of organochlorine residues from abdominal and egg fats of chickens, Ontario, Canada, 1969-1982. J Assoc Off Anal Chem, **68**: 124-129.

Frank R, Rasper J, Smout MS, & Braun HE (1988) Organochlorine residues in adipose tissues, blood and milk from Ontario residents, 1976-1985. Can J Public Health, **79**: 150-158.

Fujita M & Morikawa K (1992) Regional differences in dietary intake of environmental pollutants in Japan. J Expo Anal Environ Epidemiol, **2**(2):177-193.

Fürst P, Fürst CHR, & Wilmers K (1992) Survey of dairy products for PCDD's, PCDF's, PCB's and HCB. Chemosphere, **25**(7-10): 1039-1048.

Fürst P, Fürst C, & Wilmers K (1994) Human milk as a bioindicator for body burden of PCDDs, PCDFs, organochlorine pesticides, and PCBs. Environ Health Perspect, **102** (Suppl 1): 187-193.

Galassi S & Provini A (1981) Chlorinated pesticides and PCB contents of the two main tributaries into the Adriatic Sea. Sci Total Environ, **17**: 51-57.

Gartrell MJ, Craun JC, Podrebarac DS, & Gunderson EL (1986) Pesticides, selected elements, and other chemicals in adult total diet samples, October 1980-March 1982. J Assoc Off Anal Chem, **69**(1): 146-161.

Geike F & Parasher CD (1976a) Effect of hexachlorobenzene on some growth parameters of *Chlorella pyrenoidosa*. Bull Environ Contam Toxicol, **15**: 670-677.

Geike F & Parasher CD (1976b) Effect of hexachlorobenzene (HCB) on growth of *Tetrahymena pyriformis*. Bull Environ Contam Toxicol, **16**: 347-354.

Gilbertson M (1979) Hexachlorobenzene (HCB) in Canada. Ottawa, Ontario, Environment Canada, Environmental Protection Service (Unpublished report).

Gobas FAPC, Bedard DC, Ciborowski JJH, & Haffner GD (1989) Bioaccumulation of chlorinated hydrocarbons by mayfly (*Hexagenia limbata*) in Lake St. Clair. J Great Lakes Res, **15**: 581-588.

Gobas FAPC, McNeil EJ, Lovett-Doust L, & Haffner GD (1991) Bioconcentration of chlorinated aromatic hydrocarbons in aquatic macrophytes. Environ Sci Technol, **25:** 924-929.

Gocmen A, Peters HA, Cripps DJ, Bryan GT, & Morris CR (1989) Hexachlorobenzene episode in Turkey. Biomed Environ Sci, **2**: 36-43.

Goerz G, Bolsen K, Kalofoutis A, & Tsambaos D (1994) Influence of oral isotrentoin on hepatic and cutaneous P-450-dependent isozyme activities. Arch Dermatol Res, **286**: 104-106.

Goldey ES & Taylor DH (1992) Developmental neurotoxicity following premating maternal exposure to hexachlorobenzene in rats. Neurotoxicol Teratol, **14**: 15-21.

Goldey ES, Fisher JW, & Taylor DH (1990) Maternal transfer of hexachlorobenzene in the rat. Neurotoxicol Teratol, **12**: 562-563.

Goldstein JA, Friesen M, Scotti TM, Hickman P, Hass JR, & Bergman H (1978) Assessment of the contribution of chlorinated dibenzo-p-dioxins and dibenzofurans to hexachlorobenzene-induced toxicity, porphyria, changes in mixed function oxygenases, and histopathological changes. Toxicol Appl Pharmacol, **46**: 633-649.

Gómez-Catalán J, Planas J, To-Figueras J, Camps M, & Corbella J (1993) Organochlorine pesticide residues in the population of Catalonia (Spain). Bull Environ Contam Toxicol, **51**: 160-164.

Gómez-Catalán J, Lezaun M, To-Figueras J, & Corbella J (1995) Organochlorine residues in the adipose tissue of the population of Navarra (Spain). Bull Environ Contam Toxicol, **54**: 534-540.

Gopalaswamy UV & Aiyar AS (1986) Biotransformation and toxicity of lindane and its metabolite hexachlorobenzene in mammals. In: Morris CR & Cabral JRP ed. Hexachlorobenzene: Proceedings of an International Symposium. Lyon, International Agency for Research on Cancer, pp 267-276 (IARC Scientific Publications No. 77).

Gopalaswamy UV & Nair CKK (1992) DNA binding and mutagenicity of lindane and its metabolites. Bull Environ Contam Toxicol, **49**: 300-305.

Gorski T, Gorska E, Gorecka D, & Sikora M (1986) Hexachlorobenzene is non-genotoxic in short-term tests. In: Morris CR & Cabral JRP ed. Hexachlorobenzene: Proceedings of an International Symposium. Lyon, International Agency for Research on Cancer, pp 399-401 (IARC Scientific Publications No. 77).

Government of Canada (1993) Canadian Environmental Protection Act priority substances list assessment report: Hexachlorobenzene. Ottawa, Ontario, Environment Canada, Health and Welfare Canada, 52 pp.

Gralla EJ, Fleischman RW, Luthra YK, Hagopian M, Baker JR, Esber H, & Marcus W (1977) Toxic effects of hexachlorobenzene after daily administration to beagle dogs for one year. Toxicol Appl Pharmacol, **40**: 227-239.

Grant DL, Iverson F, Hatina GV, & Villeneuve DC (1974) Effects of hexachlorobenzene on liver porphyrin levels and microsomal enzymes in the rat. Environ Physiol Biochem, **4**: 159-165.

Grant DL, Shields JB, & Villeneuve DC (1975) Chemical (HCB) porphyria: effect of removal of sex organs in the rat. Bull Environ Contam Toxicol, **14**: 422-425.

Grant DL, Phillips WEJ, & Hatina GV (1977) Effect of hexachlorobenzene on reproduction in the rat. Arch Environ Contam Toxicol, **5**: 207-216.

Green JA, Francis JE, Wolf CR, Manson MM, & Smith AG (1989) Sexual dimorphism of cytochrome P-450 induction by hexachlorobenzene in rats. Biochem Soc Trans, **17**: 1016-1017.

Greve PA & Van Zoonen P (1990) Organochlorine pesticides and PCB's in tissues from Dutch citizens (1968-1986). Int J Environ Anal Chem, **38**: 265-277.

Griffin RA & Chou SFJ (1981) Movement of PCB's and other persistent compounds through soil. Water Sci Technol, **13**: 1153-1163.

Grimalt JO, Gomez-Belinchon JI, Llop R, & Albaiges J (1988) Water-phase distribution of hexachlorobenzene in a deltaic environment (Ebre Delta, Western Mediterranean). Chemosphere, **17**: 1893-1903.

Grimalt JO, Sunyer J, Moreno V, Amaral OC, Sala M, Rosell A, Anto JM, & Albaiges J (1994) Risk excess of soft-tissue and thyroid cancers in a community exposed to airborne organochlorinated compound mixtures with a high hexachlorobenzene content. Int J Cancer, **56**: 200-203.

Guerzoni ME, Del Cupolo L, & Ponti I (1976) [Mutagenic activity of pesticides.] Riv Sci Tech Alim Nutr Um, **6**: 161-165 (in Italian, with English summary).

Hagenmaier H, She J, & Lindig C (1992) Persistence of polychlorinated dibenzo-p-dioxins and polychlorinated dibenzofurans in contaminated soil at Maulach and Rastatt in southwest Germany. Chemosphere, **25**(7/10): 1449-1456.

Hahn ME, Gasiewicz TA, Linko P, & Goldstein JA (1988) The role of the Ah locus in hexachlorobenzene-induced porphyria. Biochem J, **254**: 245-254.

Hahn ME, Goldstein JA, Linko P, & Gasiewicz TA (1989) Interaction of hexachlorobenzene with the receptor for 2,3,7,8-tetrachlorodibenzo-p-dioxin *in vitro* and *in vivo*. Arch Biochem Biophys, **270**(1): 344-355.

Hansen LG, Dorn SB, Sundlof SM, & Vogel RS (1978) Toxicity, accumulation and depletion of hexachlorobenzene in laying chickens. J Agric Food Chem, **26**: 1369-1374.

Hansen LG, Teske RH, Sundlof SM, & Simon J (1979) Hexachlorobenzene and feline reproduction: effects of ground pork contaminated by dietary exposure or spiked with purified HCB. Vet Hum Toxicol, **21**: 248-253.

Hansen PD, Von Westernhagen H, & Rosenthal H (1985) Chlorinated hydrocarbons and hatching success in Baltic herring spring spawners. Mar Environ Res, **15:** 59-76.

Hargrave BT, Vass WP, Erickson PE, & Fowler BR (1989) Distribution of chlorinated hydrocarbon pesticides and PCBs in the Arctic Ocean. Dartmouth, NS, Department of Fisheries and Oceans, 224 pp (Canadian Technical Report of Fisheries and Aquatic Sciences No. 1644).

Harper DJ, Ridgeway IM, & Leatherland TM (1992) Concentrations of hexachlorobenzene, trichlorobenzenes and chloroform in the waters of the Forth Estuary, Scotland. Mar Pollut Bull, **24**(5): 244-249.

Haworth S, Lawlor T, Mortelmans K, Speck W, & Zeiger E (1983) *Salmonella* mutagenicity test results for 250 chemicals. Environ Mutagen, **1**(Suppl): 3-142.

Health Canada (1994) Canadian Environmental Protection Act: Human health risk assessment for priority substances. Ottawa, Ontario, Minister of Supply and Services.

Heidmann WA (1986) Hexachlorobenzene residues in selected species of land and sea birds in northern Germany. In: Morris CR & Cabral JRP ed. Hexachlorobenzene: Proceedings of an International Symposium. Lyon, International Agency for Research on Cancer, pp 223-228 (IARC Scientific Publications No. 77).

Heikes DL (1980) Residues of pentachloronitrobenzene and related compounds in peanut butter. Bull Environ Contam Toxicol, **24**: 338-343.

Heldaas SS, Langard S, & Andersen A (1989) Incidence of cancer in a cohort of magnesium production workers. Br J Ind Med, **46**: 617-623.

Hendriks AJ, Ma W-C, Brouns JJ, De Ruiter-Dijkman EM, & Gast R (1995) Modelling and monitoring organochlorine and heavy metal accumulation in soils, earthworms, and shrews in Rhine-Delta floodplains. Arch Environ Contam Toxicol, **29**: 115-127.

Herren-Freund SL & Pereira MA (1986) Carcinogenicity of by-products of disinfection in mouse and rat liver. Environ Health Perspect, **69**: 59-65.

Hill EF, Heath RG, Spann JW, & Williams JD (1975) Lethal dietary toxicities of environmental pollutants to birds. Washington, DC, US Department of Interior, Fish and Wildlife Service (Special Scientific Report — Wildlife No. 191).

Hippelein M, Kaupp H, Dörr G, & McLachlan MS (1993) Testing of a sampling system and analytical method for determination of semivolatile organic compounds in ambient air. Chemosphere, **26**: 2255-2263.

Hoff RM, Muir DCG, & Grift NP (1992) Annual cycle of polychlorinated biphenyls and organohalogen pesticides in air in southern Ontario: 1. Air concentration data. Environ Sci Technol, **26**(2): 266-275.

Holoubek I, Čáslavský J, Vancura R, Kocan A, Chovancová J, Petrik J, Drobna B, Cudlin P, & Triska J (1994) Project Tocoen: The fate of selected organic pollutants in the environment - Part XXIV. The content of PCBs and PCDDs/Fs in high-mountain soils. Toxicol Environ Chem, **45**: 189-197.

Howard PH, Boethling RS, Jarvis WF, Meylan WM, & Michalenko EM (1991) In: Taup H ed. Handbook of environmental degradation rates. Chelsea, Michigan, Lewis Publishers.

IARC (1979) Hexachlorobenzene. In: Some halogenated hydrocarbons. Lyon, International Agency for Research on Cancer, pp 155-178 (IARC Monographs on the Evaluation of the Carcinogenic Risk of Chemicals to Human, Volume 20).

IARC (1987) Hexachlorobenzene. In: Overall evaluations of carcinogenicity: An updating of IARC monographs, volumes 1 to 42. Lyon, International Agenci for Research on Cancer, pp 219-220 (IARC Monograph on the Evaluation of the Carcinogenic Risk of Chemicals to Humans, Supplement 7).

Iatropoulos MJ, Hobson W, Knauf V, & Adams HP (1976) Morphological effects of hexachlorobenzene toxicity in female rhesus monkeys. Toxicol Appl Pharmacol, **37**: 433-444.

IJC (International Joint Commission) (1989) In: Rathke DR & McRae G ed. Great Lakes surveillance: 1987 report on Great Lakes water quality. Report to the International Joint Commission, Windsor, Ontario.

Ikemoto Y, Motoba K, Suzuki T, & Uchida M (1992) Quantitative structure-activity relationships of nonspecific and specific toxicants in several organism species. Environ Toxicol Chem, **11**: 931-939.

Ingebritsen K (1986) Comparative studies on the distribution and excretion of ^{14}C-hexachlorobenzene by whole-body autoradiography. In: Morris CR & Cabral JRP ed. Hexachlorobenzene: Proceedings of an International Symposium. Lyon, International Agency for Research on Cancer, pp 277-285 (IARC Scientific Publications No. 77).

Ingebritsen K, Skaare JU, Nafstad I, & Forde M (1981) Studies on the biliary excretion and metabolites of hexachlorobenzene in the rat. Xenobiotica, **11:** 795-800.

Innes D, Muncaster B, Lazar R, Haffner D, & Hebert P (1988) Monitoring of organic contaminants using freshwater mussels. Proceedings of the Environmental Research Technology Transfer Conference, 30 November-1 December 1987 - Part B: Water quality research. Toronto, Ontario, Environment Ontario.

IPCS (1994) Environmental health criteria 170: Assessing human health risks of chemicals: The derivation of guidance values for health-based exposure limits. Geneva, World Health Organization, International Programme on Chemical Safety.

IRPTC (1993) IRPTC legal file. Geneva, United Nations Environment Programme, International Register of Potentially Toxic Chemicals.

Ishidate M Jr (1988) Data book of chromosomal aberration test *in vitro*. Amsterdam, New York, Oxford, Elsevier Science Publishers.

Jacoff FS, Scarberry R, & Rosa D (1986) Source assessment of hexachlorobenzene from the organic chemical manufacturing industry. In: Morris CR & Cabral JRP ed. Hexachlorobenzene: Proceedings of an International Symposium. Lyon, International Agency for Research on Cancer, pp 31-37 (IARC Scientific Publications No. 77). 31-37.

Jaffe R & Hites RA (1986) Anthropogenic, polyhalogenated, organic compounds in non-migratory fish from the Niagara River area and tributaries to Lake Ontario. J Great Lakes Res, **12**: 63-71.

Jansson B & Bergman A (1978) Sulfur-containing derivatives of hexachlorobenzene (HCB) - metabolites in the rat. Chemosphere, **3**: 257-268.

Jansson B, Andersson R, Asplund L, Litzen K, Nylund K, Sellström U, Uvemo U-B, Wahlberg C, Wideqvist U, Odsjö T, & Olsson M (1993) Chlorinated and brominated persistent organic compounds in biological samples from the environment. Environ Toxicol Chem, **12**: 1163-1174.

Jarrell JF, McMahon A, Villeneuve D, Franklin C, Singh A, Valli VE, & Bartlett S (1993a) Hexachlorobenzene toxicity in the monkey primordial germ cell without induced porphyria. Reprod Toxicol, **7**: 41-47.

Jarrell JF, Villeneuve D, Franklin C, Bartlett S, Wrixon W, Kohut J, & Zouves CG (1993b) Contamination of human ovarian follicular fluid and serum by chlorinated organic compounds in three Canadian cities. Can Med Assoc J, **148**(8): 1321-1327.

Jemaa Z, Sabbah S, Driss MR, & Bouguerra ML (1986) Hexachlorobenzene in Tunisian mothers' milk, cord blood and foodstuffs. In: Morris CR & Cabral JRP ed. Hexachlorobenzene: Proceedings of an International Symposium. Lyon, International Agency for Research on Cancer, pp 139-142 (IARC Scientific Publications No. 77).

Johansen HR, Becher G, Polder A, & Skaare JU (1994) Congener-specific determination of polychlorinated biphenyls and organochlorine pesticides in human milk from Norwegian mothers living in Oslo. J Toxicol Environ Health, **42**: 157-171.

Kaminsky R, Kaiser KLE, & Hites RA (1983) Fates of organic compounds from Niagara Falls dumpsites in Lake Ontario. J Great Lakes Res, **9**: 183-189.

Kan CA & Tuinstra LGM (1976) Accumulation and excretion of certain organochloride insecticides in broiler breeder hens. J Agric Food Chem, **24:** 775-778.

Kan-Do Office & Pesticides Team (1995) Accumulated pesticide and industrial chemical findings from a ten-year study of ready-to-eat foods. J Assoc Off Anal Chem, **78**(3): 614-631.

Kannan K, Tanabe S, Ramesh A, Subramanian A, & Tatsukawa R (1992a) Persistent organochlorine residues in foodstuffs from India and their implications on human dietary exposure. J Agric Food Chem, **40**: 518-524.

Kannan K, Tanabe S, Hoang Trong Quynh, Nguyen Duc Hue, & Tatsukawa R (1992b) Residue pattern and dietary intake of persistent organochlorine compounds in foodstuffs from Vietnam. Arch Environ Contam Toxicol, **22**: 367-374.

Kannan K, Falandysz J, Tanabe S, & Tatsukawa R (1993) Persistent organochlorines in Harbour Porpoises from Puck Bay, Poland. Mar Pollut Bull, **26**(3): 162-165.

Kannan K, Tanabe S, Williams RJ, & Tatsukawa R (1994) Persistant organochlorine residues in foodstuffs from Australia, Papua New Guinea and the Solomon Islands: contamination levels and human dietary exposure. Sci Total Environ, **153**: 29-49.

Kashimoto T, Takayama K, Mimura M, Miyata H, Murakami Y, & Matsumoto H (1989) PCDDs, PCDFs, PCBs, coplanar PCBs and organochlorinated pesticides in human adipose tissue in Japan. Chemosphere, **19**(1/6): 921-926.

Kasokat T, Nagel R, & Urich K (1989) Metabolism of chlorobenzene and hexachlorobenzene by the zebra fish, *Brachydanio rerio*. Bull Environ Contam Toxicol, **42**: 254-261.

Kauss PB & Hamdy YS (1985) Biological monitoring of organochlorine contaminants in the St. Clair and Detroit Rivers using introduced clams, *Elliptio complanatus*. J Great Lakes Res, **11**: 247-263.

Kelly AG & Campbell A (1994) Organochlorine contaminants in liver of cod (*Gadus morhua*) and muscle of herring (*Clupea harengus*) from Scottish waters. Mar Pollut Bull, **28**(2): 103-108.

Kemper FH (1993) Human organ specimen banking-15 years of experience. Sci Total Environ, **139-140**: 13-25.

Kennedy SW & Wigfield DC (1990) Dose-response relationships in hexachlorobenzene-induced porphyria. Biochem Pharmacol, **40**: 1381-1388.

Kennedy SW, Wigfield DC, & Fox GA (1986) The delay in polyhalogenated aromatic hydrocarbon-induced porphyria: mechanistic reality or methodological artefact? Toxicol Lett, **31**: 235-241.

Kessabi M, Elhraiki A, & Nader B (1988) Contamination of urban, industrial and continental waters by chlorinated hydrocarbon pesticides along the Mediterranean coast of Morocco. Sci Total Environ, **71**: 209-214.

Kessabi M, Abdennebi E, Laraje R, & Lhafi A (1990) Contamination of eggs, poultry liver and bovine liver and kidney by chlorinated pesticides in Morocco. Sci Total Environ, **90**: 283-287.

Khera KS (1974) Teratogenicity and dominant lethal studies on hexachlorobenzene in rats. Food Cosmet Toxicol, **12**: 471-477.

Kilikidis SD, Kamarianos AP, & Karamanlis XN (1992) Seasonal fluctuations of organochlorine compounds in the water of the Strimon River (N. Greece). Bull Environ Contam Toxicol, **49**: 375-380.

Kilzer L, Scheunert I, Geyer H, Klein W, & Korte F (1979) Laboratory screening of the volatilization rates of organic chemicals from water and soil. Chemosphere, **10**: 751-761.

Kimbrough RD & Linder RE (1974) The toxicity of technical hexachlorobenzene in the Sherman rat strain. A preliminary study. Res Commun Chem Pathol Pharmacol, **8**: 653-664.

King L & Sherbin G (1986) Point sources of toxic organics to the upper St. Clair River. Water Pollut Res J Can, **21**: 433-446.

Kitchin KT & Brown JL (1989) Biochemical studies of promoters of carcinogenesis in rat livers. Teratog Carcinog Mutagen, **9**: 273-285.

Kitchin KT, Linder RE, Scotti TM, Walsh D, Curley AO, & Svendsgaard D (1982) Offspring mortality and maternal lung pathology in female rats fed hexachlorobenzene. Toxicology, **23**: 33-39.

Kleiman de Pisarev DL, Sancovich HA, & Ferramola de Sancovich AM (1989) Enhanced thyroxine metabolism in hexachlorobenzene-intoxicated rats. J Endocrinol Invest, **12**: 767-772.

Kleiman de Pisarev DL, Del Carmen Rios de Molina M, & San Martin de Viale LC (1990) Thyroid function and thyroxine metabolism in hexachlorobenzene-induced porphyria. Biochem Pharmacol,. **39**: 817-825.

Knezovich JP & Harrison FL (1988) The bioavailability of sediment-sorbed chlorobenzenes to larvae of the midge, *Chironomus decorus*. Ecotoxicol Environ Saf, **15**: 226-241.

Kocan A, Petrik J, Drobná G, & Chovancová J (1994) Levels of PCBs and some organochlorine pesticides in the human population of selected areas of the Slovak Republic: I. Blood. Chemosphere, **29**(9/11): 2315-2325.

Kodric-Smit M, Smit Z, & Olie K (1980) Organochlorine contaminants in human milk from Slavonia Province, Yugoslavia, 1978. Pestic Monit J, **14**: 1-2.

Koeman JH, Ten Noever de Brauw MC & De Vos RH (1969) Chlorinated biphenyls in fish, mussels and birds from the river Rhine and the Netherlands coastal area. Nature (Lond), **221**: 1126-1128.

Kohler A, Harms U, & Lukas B (1986) Accumulation of organochlorines and mercury in flounder - an approach to pollution assessments. Helgol Meeresunters **40**: 431-440.

Koizumi A (1991) Experimental evidence for the possible exposure of workers to hexachlorobenzene by skin contamination. Br J Ind Med, **48:** 622-628.

Kosian P, Lemke A, Studders K, & Veith G (1981) The precision of the ASTM bioconcentration test. Duluth, Minnesota, US Environmental Protection Agency, Environmental Research Laboratory & Superior, Wisconsin, University of Wisconsin-Superior, Center for Lake Superior Environmental Studies, 24 pp (EPA 600/3-81/022).

Koss G & Koransky W (1975) Studies on the toxicology of hexachlorobenzene: I. Pharmacokinetics. Arch Toxicol, **34**: 203-212.

Koss G & Koransky W (1976) Studies on the toxicology of hexachlorobenzene. II. Identification and determination of metabolites. Arch Toxicol, **35**: 107-114.

Koss G & Koransky W (1978) Pentachlorophenol in different species of vertebrates after administration of hexachlorobenzene and pentachlorobenzene. In: Ranga Rao K ed. Pentachlorophenol. New York, London, Plenum Press, pp 131-137.

Koss G & Manz D (1976) Residues of hexachlorobenzene in wild mammals of Germany. Bull Environ Contam Toxicol, **15**: 189-191.

Koss G, Strik JJTWA, & Kan CA (1978) Metabolites of hexachlorobenzene in the excreta of different animal species. Excerpta Med Int Congress, **440**: 211-212.

Krauthacker B (1993) Organochlorine pesticides and polychlorinated biphenyls (PCBs) in human serum collected from the general population from Zagreb (1985-1990). Bull Environ Contam Toxicol, **50**: 8-11.

Krishnan K, Brodeur J, & Charbonneau M (1991) Development of an experimental model for the study of hexachlorobenzene-induced hepatic porphyria in the rat. Toxicol Appl Pharmacol, **17**: 433-441.

Krishnan K, Brodeur J, Plaa GL, & Charbonneau M (1992) Modulation of hexachlorobenzene-induced hepatic porphyria by methyl isobutyl ketone in the rat. Toxicol Lett, **61**: 167-174.

Kuehl DW & Butterworth B (1994) A national study of chemical residues in fish: III. Study results. Chemosphere, **29**(3): 523-535.

Kuehl DW, Leonard EN, Butterworth BC, & Johnson KL (1983) Polychlorinated chemical residues in fish from major watersheds near the Great Lakes, 1979. Environ Int, **9**: 293-299.

Kuhnlein HV, Receveur O, Muir DCG, Chan HM, & Soueida R (1995) Arctic indigenous women consume greater than acceptable levels of organochlorines. J Nutr, **125**: 2501-2510.

Kuiper-Goodman T, Grant DL, Moodle CA, Korsrud GO, & Munro IC (1977) Subacute toxicity of hexachlorobenzene in the rat. Toxicol Appl Pharmacol, **40**: 529-549.

Kuroda Y (1986) Genetic and chemical factors affecting chemical mutagenesis in cultured mammalian cells. In: Antimutagenesis and anticarcinogenesis mechanisms. New York, London, Plenum Press, pp 359-375.

Lambrecht RW, Erturk E, Grunden EE, Headley DB, Peters HA, Morris CR, & Bryan GT (1982a) Renal toxicity and tumorigenicity of hexachlorobenzene (HCB) in rats (R). Proc Am Assoc Cancer Res, **23**: 54 (Abstract).

Lambrecht RW, Erturk E, Grunden E, Headley DB, Morris CR, Peters HA, & Bryan GT (1982b) Hepatotoxicity and tumorigenicity of hexachlorobenzene (HCB) in Syrian golden hamsters (H) after subchronic administration. Fed Proc, **41**: 329 (Abstract).

Lambrecht RW, Ertürk E, Grunden EE, Peters HA, Morris CR, & Bryan GT (1983a) Hepatocarcinogenicity of chronically administered hexachlorobenzene in rats. Fed Proc, **42**: 786 (Abstract).

Lambrecht RW, Ertürk E, Grunden EE, Peters HA, Morris CR, & Bryan GT (1983b) Renal tumors in rats chronically exposed to hexachlorobenzene (HCB). Proc Am Assoc Cancer Res, **24**: 59 (Abstract).

Lambrecht RW, Sinclair PR, Bement WJ, Sinclair JF, Carpenter HM, Buhler DR, Urquhart AJ, & Elder GH (1988) Hepatic uroporphyrin accumulation and uroporphyrinogen decarboxylase activity in cultured chick-embryo hepatocytes and in Japanese quail (*Coturnix coturnix japonica*) and mice treated with polyhalogenated aromatic hydrocarbons. Biochem J, **253**: 131-138.

Lamparski LL, Langhorst ML, Nestrick TJ, & Cutie S (1980) Gas-liquid chromatographic determination of chlorinated benzenes and phenols in selected biological matrices. J Assoc Off Anal Chem, **63**(1): 27-32.

Landrum PF (1989) Bioavailability and toxicokinetics of polycyclic aromatic hydrocarbons sorbed to sediment for the amphipod *Pontoporeia hoyi*. Environ Sci Technol, **23**: 588-595.

Lane DA, Schroeder WH, & Johnson ND (1992a) On the spatial and temporal variations in atmospheric concentrations of hexachlorobenzene and hexachlorocyclohexane isomers at several locations in the province of Ontario, Canada. Atmos Environ, **26A**: 31-42.

Lane DA, Johnson ND, Hanley MJJ, Schroeder WH, & Ord DT (1992b) Gas- and particle-phase concentrations of α-hexachlorocyclohexane, γ-hexachlorocyclohexane, and hexachlorobenzene in Ontario air. Environ Sci Technol, **26**: 126-133.

Langhorst ML & Nestrick TJ (1979) Determination of chlorobenzenes in air and biological samples by gas chromatography with photoionization detection. Anal Chem, **51**(12): 2018-2025.

Larsen BR, Turrio-Baldassarri L, Nilsson T, Iacovella N, Di Domenico A, Montagna M, & Facchetti S (1994) Toxic PCB congeners and organochlorine pesticides in Italian human milk. Ecotoxicol Environ Saf, **28**: 1-13.

Laseter JL, Bartell CK, Laska AL, Holmquist DG, Condie DB, Brown JW, & Evans RL (1976) An ecological study of hexachlorobenzene (HCB). New Orleans, University of New Orleans, Department of Biological Sciences (Prepared for the US Environmental Protection Agency, Office of Toxic Substances, Washington) (EPA 560/6-76-009).

Laska AL, Bartell C, & Laseter JL (1976) Distribution of hexachlorobenzene and hexachlorobutadiene in water, soil, and selected aquatic organisms along the lower Mississippi River, Louisiana. Bull Environ Contam Toxicol, **15**: 535-542.

Leger DA (1991) Environmental concentrations of hexachlorobenzene in Atlantic Canada. Moncton, New Brunswick, Environment Canada, Inland Waters Directorate.

Leoni V & D'Arca SU (1976) Experimental data and critical review of the occurrence of hexachlorobenzene in the Italian environment. Sci Total Environ, **5**: 253-272.

Lewis RJ (1992) Sax's dangerous properties of industrial materials, 8th ed. New York, Van Nostrand Reinhold Company.

Lewis RG & MacLeod KE (1982) Portable sampler for pesticides and semivolatile industrial organic chemicals in air. Anal Chem, **54**: 310-315.

Ligocki MP, Leuenberger C, & Pankow JF (1985) Trace organic compounds in rain: II. Gas scavenging of neutral organic compounds. Atmos Environ, **19**: 1609-1617.

Lilienthal H, Benthe C, Heinzow B, & Winneke G (1996) Impairment of schedule-controlled behavior by pre- and postnatal exposure to hexachlorobenzene in rats. Arch Toxicol, **70**: 174-181.

Linko P, Yeowell HN, Gasiewicz TA, & Goldstein JA (1986) Induction of cytochrome P-450 isozymes by hexachlorobenzene in rats and aromatic hydrocarbon (Ah)-responsive mice. J Biochem Toxicol, **1**: 95-107.

Loose LD (1982) Macrophage induction of T-suppressor cells in pesticide-exposed and protozoan-infected mice. Environ Health Perspect, **43**: 89-97.

Loose LD, Silkworth JB, Charbonneau T, & Blumenstock F (1981) Environmental chemical-induced macrophage dysfunction. Environ Health Perspect, **39**: 79-92.

Lopez-Avila V, Northcutt R, Onstot J, Wickham M, & Billets S (1983) Determination of 51 priority organic compounds after extraction from standard reference materials. Anal Chem, **55**(6): 881-889.

Lu P & Metcalf RL (1975) Environmental fate and biodegradability of benzene derivatives as studied in a model ecosystem. Environ Health Perspect, **10:** 269-284.

Ludwicki JK & Góralczyk K (1994) Organochlorine pesticides and PCBs in human adipose tissues in Poland. Bull Environ Contam Toxicol, **52**: 400-403.

Lunde G & Bjorseth A (1977) Human blood samples as indicators of occupational exposure to persistent chlorinated hydrocarbons. Sci Total Environ, **8**(3): 241-246.

Lunde G & Ofstad EB (1976) Determination of fat-soluble chorinated compounds in fish. Z Anal Chem, **282**: 395-399.

McCarty LS, MACKAY D, Smith AD, Ozburn GW, & Dixon DG (1992a) Residue-based interpretation of toxicity and bioconcentration QSARs from aquatic bioassays: Neutral narcotic organics. Environ Toxicol Chem, **11**: 917-930.

McCarty LS, Ozburn GW, Smith AD, & Dixon DG (1992b) Toxicokinetic modeling of mixtures of organic chemicals. Environ Toxicol Chem, **11**: 1037-1047.

Mack GA & Stanley J (1985) The national human adipose tissue survey. Washington, DC, US Environmental Protection Agency, Office of Pesticides and Toxic Substances (Report No. NHATS-ST-01).

Mackay D, Shiu WY, & Ma KC (1992) Illustrated handbook of physical-chemical properties and environmental fate for organic chemicals - Volume I: Monoaromatic hydrocarbons, chlorobenzenes, and PCBs. Chelsea, Michigan, Lewis Publishers.

McLeese DW & Metcalfe CD (1980) Toxicities of eight organochlorine compounds in sediment and seawater to *Crangon septemspinosa*. Bull Environ Contam Toxicol, **25**: 921-928.

MAFF (Ministry of Agriculture, Fisheries and Food) (1992) Report of the working party on pesticide residues: 1988-1990. London, Her Majesty's Stationery Office (Food Surveillance Paper No. 34).

MAFF/HSE (Ministry of Agriculture, Fisheries and Food/Health and Safety Executive) (1994) Report of the working party on pesticide residues, 1993 - Supplement to the pesticides register. London, Her Majesty's Stationery Office.

Mansour M, Scheunert I, Viswanathan R, & Korte F (1986) Assessment of the persistence of hexachlorobenzene in the ecosphere. In: Morris CR & Cabral JRP ed. Hexachlorobenzene: Proceedings of an International Symposium. Lyon, International Agency for Research on Cancer, pp 53-59 (IARC Scientific Publications No. 77).

Marlow DA (1986) Hexachlorobenzene exposure in the production of chlorophenols. In: Morris CR & Cabral JRP ed. Hexachlorobenzene: Proceedings of an International Symposium. Lyon, International Agency for Research on Cancer, pp 161-169 (IARC Scientific Publications No. 77).

Mehendale HM, Fields M, & Matthews HB (1975) Metabolism and effects of hexachlorobenzene on hepatic microsomal enzymes in the rat. J Agric Food Chem, **23**: 261-265.

Mendoza CE, Grant DL, & Shields JB (1975) Body burden of hexachlorobenzene in suckling rats and its effects on various organs and on liver porphyrin accumulation. Environ Physiol Biochem, **5**: 460-464.

Mendoza CE, Collins B, Shields JB, & Laver GW (1977) Hexachlorobenzene residues and effects on esterase activities in pre-weanling rats after a reciprocal transfer between HCB-treated and control dams. Arch Toxicol, **38**: 191-199.

Mendoza CE, Collins BT, Shields JB, & Laver GW (1978) Effects of hexachlorobenzene or hexabromobenzene on body and organ weights of preweanling rats after a reciprocal transfer between the treated and control dams. J Agric Food Chem, **26**: 941-945.

Mendoza CE, Shields JB, & Laver GW (1979) Comparison of the porphyrinogenic activity of hexabromobenzene and hexachlorobenzene in primiparous Wistar rats. Bull Environ Contam Toxicol, **21**: 358-364.

Mes J (1990) Trends in the levels of some chlorinated hydrocarbon residues in adipose tissue of Canadians. Environ Pollut, **65**: 269-278.

Mes J (1992) Organochlorine residues in human blood and biopsy fat and their relationship. Bull Environ Contam Toxicol, **48**: 815-820.

Mes J & Davies DJ (1979) Presence of polychlorinated biphenyl and organochlorine pesticide residues and the absence of polychlorinated terphenyls in Canadian human milk samples. Bull Environ Contam Toxicol, **21**: 381-387.

Mes J & Malcolm S (1992) Comparison of chlorinated hydrocarbon residues in human populations from the Great Lakes and other regions of Canada. Chemosphere, **25**(3): 417-424.

Mes J, Campbell DS, Robinson RN, & Davies DJA (1977) Polychlorinated biphenyl and organochlorine pesticide residues in adipose tissue of Canadians - 1977. Bull Environ Contam Toxicol, **17**: 196-203.

Mes J, Davies DJ, & Turton D (1982) Polychlorinated biphenyl and other chlorinated hydrocarbon residues in adipose tissue of Canadians. Bull Environ Contam Toxicol, **28**: 97-104.

Mes J, Davies DJ, Turton D, & Sun W-F (1986) Levels and trends of chlorinated hydrocarbon contaminants in the breast milk of Canadian women. Food Addit Contam, **3**: 313-322.

Mes J, Marchand L, & Davies DJ (1990) Organochlorine residues in adipose tissue of Canadians. Bull Environ Contam Toxicol, **45**: 681-688.

Mes J, Davies DJ, Doucet J, Weber D, & McMullen E (1993) Levels of chlorinated hydrocarbon residues in Canadian human breast milk and their relationship to some characteristics of the donors. Food Addit Contam, **10**(4): 429-441.

Mill T & Haag W (1986) The environmental fate of hexachlorobenzene. In: Morris CR & Cabral JRP ed. Hexachlorobenzene: Proceedings of an International Symposium. Lyon, International Agency for Research on Cancer, pp 61-66 (IARC Scientific Publications No. 77).

Moksnes MT & Norheim G (1986) Levels of chlorinated hydrocarbons and composition of PCB in herring gull *Larus argentatus* eggs collected in Norway in 1969 compared to 1979-81. Environ Pollut, **11**: 109-116.

Mollenhauer HH, Johnson JH, Younger RL, & Clark DE (1975) Ultrastructural changes in liver of the rat fed hexachlorobenzene. Am J Vet Res, **36**: 1777-1781.

Mollenhauer HH, Johnston JH, Younger RL, & Clark DE (1976) A unique intracellular aberration related to hexachlorobenzene ingestion. Am J Vet Res, **37**: 847-850.

Morita M, Mimura S, & Yagyu H (1975) A systematic determination of chlorinated benzenes in human adipose tissue. Environ Pollut, **9**: 175-179.

Morley A, Geary D, & Harben F (1973) Hexachlorobenzene pesticides and porphyria. Med J Aust, **1**: 565.

Morosini M, Schreltmüller J, Reuter U, & Ballschmiter K (1993) Correlation between C-6/C-14 chlorinated hydrocarbons levels in the vegetation and in the boundary layer of the troposphere. Environ Sci Technol, **27**: 1517-1523.

Muir DCG, Wagemann R, Grift NP, Norstrom RJ, Simon M, & Lien J (1988) Organochlorine chemical and heavy metal contaminants in white-beaked dolphins (*Lagenorhynchus albirostris*) and pilot whales (*Globicephala melaena*) from the coast of Newfoundland, Canada. Arch Environ Contam Toxicol, **17**: 613-629.

Muir DCG, Grift NP, Lockhart WL, Wilkinson P, Billeck BN, & Brunskill GJ (1995) Spatial trends and historical profiles of organochlorine pesticides in Arctic lake sediments. Sci Total Environ, **160/161**: 447-457.

Müller MD (1982) [Hexachlorobenzene in Switzerland: Measurement and background of environmental contamination.] Chimia, **36**(11): 437-445 (in German).

Mumma CF & Lawless EW (1975) Survey of industrial processing data. Task I: Hexachlorobenzene and hexachlorobutadiene pollution from chlorocarbon processes. Washington, DC, US Environmental Protection Agency, Office of Toxic Substances (EPA 560/3-75-003).

Muncaster BW, Innes DJ, Hebert PDN, & Haffner GD (1989) Patterns of organic contaminant accumulation by freshwater mussels in the St. Clair River, Ontario. J Great Lakes Res, **15**: 645-653.

Murray HE, Neff GS, Hrung Y, & Giam CS (1980) Determination of benzo(a)pyrene, hexachlorobenzene and pentachlorophenol in oysters from Galveston Bay, Texas. Bull Environ Contam Toxicol, **25**(4): 663-667.

Mussalo-Rauhamaa H, Pyysalo H, & Antervo K (1988) Relation between the content of organochlorine compounds in Finnish human milk and characteristics of the mothers. J Toxicol Environ Health, **25**: 1-19.

Nair A & Pillai MKK (1989) Monitoring of hexachlorobenzene residues in Delhi and Faridabad, India. Bull Environ Contam Toxicol, **42**: 682-686.

Nash RG & Gish TJ (1989) Halogenated pesticide volatilization and dissipation from soil under controlled conditions. Chemosphere, **18**: 2353-2362.

Nebecker AV, Griffis WL, Wise CM, Hopkins E, & Barbitta JA (1989) Survival, reproduction and bioconcentration in invertebrates and fish exposed to hexachlorobenzene. Environ Toxicol Chem, **8**: 601-611.

Needham LL, Burse VW, Head SL, Korver MP, McClure PC, Andrews JS Jr, Rowley DL, Sung J, & Kahn SE (1990) Adipose tissue/serum partitioning of chlorinated hydrocarbon pesticides in humans. Chemosphere, **20**: 975-980.

Newton KG & Greene NC (1972) Organochlorine pesticide residue levels in human milk -Victoria, Australia - 1970. Pestic Monit J, **6**(1): 4-8.

NHW (National Health and Welfare) (1987) Nutrient value of some common foods. Ottawa, Ontario, Health Services and Promotion Branch/Health Protection Branch.

Niimi AJ & Cho CY (1981) Elimination of hexachlorobenzene (HCB) by rainbow trout (*Salmo gairdneri*), and an examination of its kinetics in Lake Ontario salmonids. Can J Fish Aquat Sci, **38:** 1350-1356.

Niimi AJ & Oliver BG (1989) Distribution of polychlorinated biphenyl congeners and other halocarbons in whole fish and muscle among Lake Ontario salmonids. Environ Sci Technol, **23**: 83-88.

NIOSH (1985) Registry of toxic effects of chemical substances, 1983-1984 - Cumulative supplement to the 1981-1982 edition. Cincinnati, Ohio, National Institute for Occupational Safety and Health.

Noble DG & Elliott JE (1986) Environmental contaminants in Canadian seabirds, 1968-1984: Trends and effects. Ottawa, Ontario, Canadian Wildlife Service (Technical Report Series No. 13).

Noble DG, Elliott JE, & Shutt L (1992) Contaminants in Canadian raptors, 1965-1988. Ottawa, Ontario, Canadian Wildlife Service (Technical Report Series No. 91).

Norén K (1983a) Levels of organochlorine contaminants in human milk in relation to the dietary habits of the mothers. Acta Paediatr Scand, **72**: 811-816.

Norén K (1983b) Some aspects of the determination of organochlorine contaminants in human milk. Arch Environ Contam Toxicol, **12**: 277-283.

Norén K (1988) Changes in the levels of organochlorine pesticides, polychlorinated biphenyls, dibenzo-p-dioxins and dibenzofurans in human milk from Stockholm, 1972-1985. Chemosphere, **17**(1): 39-49.

Norén K (1993) Contemporary and retrospective investigations of human milk in the trend studies of organochlorine contaminants in Sweden. Sci Total Environ, **139/140**: 347-355.

Norstrom RJ, Simon M, & Muir DCG (1990) Polychlorinated dibenzo-p-dioxins and dibenzofurans in marine mammals in the Canadian north. Environ Pollut, **66**: 1-19.

NTP (1994) Seventh annual report on carcinogens. Summary, 1994. Research Triangle Park North Carolina, US Department of Health and Human Services, National Toxicology Program.

Ockner RK & Schmid R (1961) Acquired porphyria in man and rat due to hexachlorobenzene intoxication. Nature (Lond), **189**: 499.

Oehme M & Stray H (1982) Quantitative determination of ultra-traces of chlorinated compounds in high-volume air samples from the Arctic using polyurethane foam as collection medium. Fresenius Z Anal Chem, **311**: 665-673.

Oliver BG (1984a) Distribution and pathways of some chlorinated benzenes in the Niagara River and Lake Ontario. Water Pollut Res J Can, **19**: 47-59.

Oliver BG (1984b) Uptake of chlorinated organics from anthropogenically contaminated sediments by oligochaete worms. Can J Fish Aquat Sci, **41**: 878-883.

Oliver BG (1987) Partitioning relationships for chlorinated organics between water and particulates in the St. Clair, Detroit and Niagara Rivers. In: Kaiser LLE ed. QSAR in environmental toxicology - II. Boston, Massachussetts, D. Reidel Publishing Co., pp 251-260.

Oliver BG & Bourbonniere RA (1985) Chlorinated contaminants in surficial sediments of Lakes Huron, St. Clair, and Erie: Implications regarding sources along the St. Clair and Detroit rivers. J Great Lakes Res, **11**: 366-372.

Oliver BG & Carey JH (1986) Photodegradation of wastes and pollutants in aquatic environment. In: Pelizzetti E & Serpo N ed. Homogenous and heterogenous photocatalysis. Boston, Massachussetts, D. Reidel Publishing Co., pp 629-650.

Oliver BG & Charlton MN (1984) Chlorinated organic contaminants on settling particulates in the Niagara River vicinity of Lake Ontario. Environ Sci Technol, **18**: 903-908.

Oliver BG & Kaiser KLE (1986) Chlorinated organics in nearshore waters and tributaries of the St. Clair River. Water Pollut Res J Can, **21**: 344-350.

Oliver BG & Nicol KD (1982) Chlorobenzenes in sediments, water, and selected fish from Lakes Superior, Huron, Erie, and Ontario. Environ Sci Technol, **16**: 532-536.

Oliver BG & Niimi AJ (1988) Trophodynamic analysis of polychlorinated biphenyl congeners and other chlorinated hydrocarbons in the Lake Ontario ecosystem. Environ Sci Technol, **22**: 388-397.

Oliver BG & Pugsley CW (1986) Chlorinated contaminants in St. Clair River sediments. Water Pollut Res J Can, **21**: 368-379.

Oliver BG, Charlton MN, & Durham RW (1989) Distribution, redistribution, and geochronology of polychlorinated biphenyl congeners and other chlorinated hydrocarbons in Lake Ontario sediments. Environ Sci Technol, **23**: 200-208.

OMAF/OME (Ontario Ministry of Agriculture and Food/Ontario Ministry of the Environment) (1988) Polychlorinated dibenzo-p-dioxins and polychlorinated dibenzofurans and other organochlorine contaminants in food. Toronto, Ontario Ministry of Agriculture and Food and Ministry of the Environment (Report prepared by the Joint OMAF/OME Toxics in Food Steering Committee).

Ostfeldt P, Gustavson K, Jansson B, Jonsson P, Miettinen V, Ringstad O, & Wesén C (1994) Halogenated organic compounds in the marine environment 1989-1990. Copenhagen, Nordic Council of Ministers, 124 pp (TemaNord 1994:591).

Parrish PR, Cook GH, & Patrick JM Jr (1974) Effects on several estuarine animals. In: Rogers WA ed. Proceedings of the 28th Annual Conference, White Sulphur Springs, West Virginia, 17-20 November 1974. Sulphur Springs, West Virginia, Southeastern Association of Game and Fish Commissioners.

Patton GW, Hinckley DA, Walla MD, & Bidleman TF (1989) Airborne organochlorines in the Canadian High Arctic. Tellus, **41B**: 243-255.

Peakall DB, Noble DG, Elliott JE, Somers JD, & Erickson G (1990) Environmental contaminants in Canadian peregrine falcons, *Falco peregrinus*: A toxicological assessment. Can Field-Nat, **104**: 244-254.

Pearce PA, Elliott JE, Peakall DB, & Norstrom RJ (1989) Organochlorine contaminants in eggs of seabirds in the Northwest Atlantic, 1968-1984. Environ Pollut, **56**: 217-235.

Pereira MA, Herren SL, Britt AL, & Khoury MM (1982) Sex difference in enhancement of GGTase-positive foci by hexachlorobenzene and lindane in rat liver. Cancer Lett, **15**: 95-101.

Persoone G & Uyttersprot G (1975) The influence of inorganic and organic pollutants on the rate of reproduction of a marine hypotrichous ciliate: *Euplotes vannus* Muller. Rev Int Océanogr méd, **37-38**: 125-151.

Peters HA (1976) Hexachlorobenzene poisoning in Turkey. Fed Proc, **35**: 2400-2403.

Peters HA, Johnson SAM, Cam S, Oral S, Müftü Y, & Ergene T (1966) Hexachlorobenzene-induced porphyria: effect of chelation on the disease, porphyrin and metal metabolism. Am J Med Sci, **251**: 314-322.

Peters HA, Gocmen A, Cripps DJ, Bryan GT, & Dogramaci I (1982) Epidemiology of hexachlorobenzene-induced porphyria in Turkey: clinical and laboratory follow-up after 25 years. Arch Neurol, **39**: 744-749.

Peters HA, Cripps DJ, Gocmen A, Ertürk E, Bryan GT, & Morris CR (1986) Neurotoxicity of hexachlorobenzene-induced porphyria turcica. In: Morris CR & Cabral JRP ed. Hexachlorobenzene: Proceedings of an International Symposium. Lyon, International Agency for Research on Cancer, pp 575-579 (IARC Scientific Publications No. 77).

Peterson R & Ray S (1987) Organochlorine residues in brook trout and yellow perch from New Brunswick and Nova Scotia (Canada) lakes. Water Pollut Res J Can, **22**: 352-364.

Phelps DK, Pruell RJ, & Lake JL (1986) Hexachlorobenzene in selected marine samples: an environmental perspective. In: Morris CR & Cabral JRP ed. Hexachlorobenzene: Proceedings of an International Symposium. Lyon, International Agency for Research on Cancer, pp 121-130 (IARC Scientific Publications No. 77).

Proulx G, Weseloh DV, Elliott JE, Teeple S, Anghern PAM, & Mineau P (1987) Organochlorine and PCB residues in Lake Erie mink populations. Bull Environ Contam Toxicol, **39**: 939-944.

Quinlivan S, Ghassemi M, & Santy M (1975) Survey of methods used to control wastes containing hexachlorobenzene. Washington, DC, US Environmental Protection Agency, Office of Solid Waste Management Programs (EPA 530/SW-120c).

Quinsey PM, Donohue DC, & Ahokas JT (1995) Persistence of organochlorines in breast milk of women in Victoria, Australia. Food Chem Toxicol, **33**(1): 49-56.

Ray LE, Murray HR, & Giam CS (1983a) Analysis of water and sediment from the Nueces Estuary/Corpus Christi Bay (Texas) for selected organic pollutants. Chemosphere, **12**: 1039-1045.

Ray LE, Murray HE, & Giam CS (1983b) Organic pollutants in marine samples from Portland, Maine. Chemosphere, **12**: 1031-1038.

Renner G (1988) Hexachlorobenzene and its metabolism. Toxicol Environ Chem, **18**: 51-78.

Richter E & Schäfer SG (1981) Intestinal excretion of hexachlorobenzene. Arch Toxicol, **47**: 233-239.

Rios de Molina MC, Wainstok de Calmanovici R, & San Martin de Viale LC (1980) Investigations on the presence of porphyrinogen carboxy-lyase inhibitor in the liver of rats intoxicated with hexachlorobenzene. Int J Biochem, **12**: 1027-1032.

Rippen G & Frank R (1986) Estimation of hexachlorobenzene pathways from the technosphere into the environment. In: Morris CR & Cabral JRP ed. Hexachlorobenzene: Proceedings of an International Symposium. Lyon, International Agency for Research on Cancer, pp 45-52 (IARC Scientific Publications No. 77).

RIWA (1993) Rapport annuel 1993 de l'Association des Services d'Eau du Rhin et de la Meuse, Annex 11. Amsterdam, Secrétariat de l'Association des Services d'Eau du Rhin et de la Meuse.

Rizzardini M & Smith AG (1982) Sex differences in the metabolism of hexachlorobenzene by rats and the development of porphyria in females. Biochem Pharmacol, **31**: 3543-3548.

Rizzardini M, Graziani A, Carugo C, & Cantoni L (1988) Investigations on the role of free radical processes in hexachlorobenzene-induced porphyria in mice. J Biochem Toxicol, **3**: 33-46.

Rizzardini M, Cantoni L, Villa P, & Ubezio P (1990) Biochemical, morphological and flow-cytometric evaluation of the effects of hexachlorobenzene on rat liver. Cell Biol Toxicol, **6**: 185-203.

Robinson PE, Mack GA, Remmers J, Levy R, & Mohadjer L (1990) Trends of PCB, hexachlorobenzene, and ß-benzene hexachloride levels in the adipose tissue of the U.S. population. Environ Res, **53**: 175-192.

Rogers HR, Crathorne B, & Leatherland TM (1989) Occurrence of chlorobenzene isomers in the water column of a UK estuary. Mar Pollut Bull, **20**: 276-281.

Rozman K, Rozman T, & Greim H (1981) Enhanced fecal elimination of stored hexachlorobenzene from rats and rhesus monkeys by hexadecane or mineral oil. Toxicology, **22**: 33-44.

Rozman K, Gorski JR, Rozman P, & Parkinson A (1986) Reduced serum thyroid hormone levels in hexachlorobenzene-induced porphyria. Toxicol Lett, **30**: 71-78.

Rumsby PC, Evans JG, Phillimore HE, Carthew P, & Smith AG (1992) Search for Ha-*ras* codon 51 mutations in liver tumours caused by hexachlorobenzene and Aroclor 1254 in C57BL/10ScSn mice with iron overload. Carcinogenesis, **13**: 1917-1920.

Rush GF, Smith JH, Maita K, Bleavins M, Aulerich RJ, Ringer RK, & Hook JB (1983) Perinatal hexachlorobenzene toxicity in the mink. Environ Res, **31**: 116-124.

Russell RW & Gobas FAPC (1989) Calibration of the freshwater mussel, *Elliptio complanata*, for quantitative biomonitoring of hexachlorobenzene and octachlorostyrene in aquatic systems. Bull Environ Contam Toxicol, **43**: 576-582.

Salisbury CDC, Fesser ACE, MacNeil JD, & Patterson JR (1992) Trace metal and pesticide levels in muskoxen from Victoria Island, Northwest Territories, Canada. Intern. J Environ Chem, **48**: 209-215.

Sanborn JR, Childers WF, & Hansen LG (1977) Uptake and elimination of [^{14}C] hexachlorobenzene (HCB) by the green sunfish, *Lepomis cyanellus* Raf., after feeding contaminated food. J Agric Food Chem, **25**: 551-553.

Schechter A, Fürst P, Krüger C, Meemken H-A, Groebel W, & Constable JD (1989a) Levels of polychlorinated dibenzofurans, dibenzodioxins, PCBs, DDT and DDE, hexachlorobenzene, dieldrin, hexachlorocyclohexanes and oxychlordane in human breast milk from the United States, Thailand, Vietnam, and Germany. Chemosphere, **18**: 445-454.

Schechter A, Mes J, & Davies D (1989b) Polychlorinated biphenyl (PCB), DDT, DDE and hexachlorobenzene (HCB) and PCDD/PCDF isomer levels in various organs in autopsy tissue from North American patients. Chemosphere, **18**: 811-818.

Scheufler E & Rozman KK (1984) Comparative decontamination of hexachlorobenzene-exposed rats and rabbits by hexadecane. J Toxicol Environ Health, **14**: 353-362.

Scheunert I, Marra C, Viswanatha R, Klein WK, & Korte F (1983) Fate of hexachlorobenzene-^{14}C in wheat plants and soil under outdoor conditions. Chemosphere, **12**: 843-858.

Scheunert I, Topp E, Schmitzer J, Klein W, & Korte F (1985) Formation and fate of bound residues of [^{14}C] benzene and [^{14}C] chlorobenzene in soil and plants. Ecotoxicol Environ Saf, **9**: 159-170.

Schielen P, Schoo W, Tekstra J, Oostermeijer HHA, Seinen W, & Bloksma N (1993) Autoimmmune effects of hexachlorobenzene in the rat. Toxicol Appl Pharmacol, **122**: 233-243.

Schielen P, Den Besten C, Vos JG, Van Bladeren PJ, Seinen W, & Bloksma N (1995) Immune effects of hexachlorobenzene in the rat: role of metabolism in a 13-week feeding study. Toxicol Appl Pharmacol, **131**: 37-43.

Schmid R (1960) Cutaneous porphyria in Turkey. N Engl J Med, **263**: 397-398.

Schmitt CJ, Zaijcek JL, & Peterman PH (1990) National Contaminant Biomonitoring Program: residues of organochlorine chemicals in U.S. freshwater fish, 1976-1984. Arch. Environ Toxicol, **19**: 748-781.

Schuler W, Brunn H, & Manz D (1985) Pesticides and polychlorinated biphenyls in fish from the Lahn River. Bull Environ Contam Toxicol, **34**: 608-616.

Schuytema G, Krawczyk DF, Griffis WL, Nebeker AV, & Robideaux ML (1990) Hexachlorobenzene uptake by fathead minnows and macroinvertebrates in recirculating sediment/water systems. Arch Environ Contam Toxicol, **19**: 1-9.

Schwarzenbach RP, Giger W, Hoehn E, & Schneider JK (1983) Behaviour of organic compounds during infiltration of river water to groundwater. Field studies. Environ Sci Technol, **17**: 472-479.

Selden A, Jacobson G, Berg P, & Axelson O (1989) Hepatocellular carcinoma and exposure to hexachlorobenzene: a case report. Br J Ind Med, **46**: 138-140.

Shirai T, Miyata Y, Nakanishi K, Murasaki G, & Ito N (1978) Hepatocarcinogenicity of polychlorinated terphenyl (PCT) in ICR mice and its enhancement by hexachlorobenzene. Cancer Lett, **4**: 271-275.

Siekel P, Chalupa I, Beno J, Blasko M, Novotny J, & Burian J (1991) A genotoxicological study of hexachlorobenzene and pentachloroanisole. Teratog Carcinog Mutagen, **11**: 55-60.

Simon GS, Tardiff RG, & Borzelleca JF (1979) Failure of hexachlorobenzene to induce dominant lethal mutations in the rat. Toxicol Appl Pharmacol, **47**: 415-419.

Sims DE, Singh A, Donald A, Jarrell J, & Villeneuve DC (1991) Alteration of primate ovary surface epithelium by exposure to hexachlorobenzene: a quantitative study. Histol Histopathol, **6**: 525-529.

Singh A, Friesen D, Jarrel J, & Villeneuve DC (1990a) Hexachlorobenzene toxicity in the monkey ovary: I. Ultrastructure induced by low (0.1 mg/kg) dose exposure. In: Proceedings of the XIIth International Congress for Electron Microscopy, Seattle, Washington - Volume 2: Analytical sciences, San Francisco, California, San Francisco Press, Inc., pp 282-283.

Singh A, Sims DE, Jarrell J, & Villeneuve DC (1990b) Hexachlorobenzene toxicity in the monkey ovary: II. Ultrastructure induced by medium (1.0 mg/kg) dose exposure. Anal Environ Toxicants, **13**: 435-438.

Singh A, Dykeman A, Jarrell J, & Villeneuve DC (1991) Hexachlorobenzene toxicity in the monkey ovary: III. Ultrastructure induced by high (10 mg/kg) dose exposure. In: Proceedings of the 49th Annual Meeting of the Electron Microscopy Society of America. San Francisco, California, San Francisco Press, Inc.

Skåre JU, Stenersen J, Kveseth N, & Polder A (1985) Time trends of organochlorine chemical residues in seven sedentary marine fish species from a Norwegian fjord during the period 1972-1982. Arch Environ Contam Toxicol, **14**: 33-41.

Skaare JU, Markussen NH, Norheim G, Haugen S, & Holt G (1990) Levels of polychlorinated biphenyls, organochlorine pesticides, mercury, cadmium, copper, selenium, arsenic, and zinc in the harbour seal, *Phoca vitulina*, in Norwegian waters. Environ Pollut, **66**: 309-324.

Smith AG & Cabral JR (1980) Liver-cell tumours in rats fed hexachlorobenzene. Cancer Lett, **11**: 169-172.

Smith AG & De Matteis F (1990) Oxidative injury mediated by the hepatic cytochrome P-450 system in conjunction with cellular iron. Effects on the pathway of haem biosynthesis. Xenobiotica, **29**(9): 865-877.

Smith AG & Francis JE (1983) Synergism of iron and hexachlorobenzene inhibits hepatic uroporphyrinogen decarboxylase in inbred mice. Biochem J, **214**: 909-913.

Smith VE, Spurr JM, Filkins JC, & Jones JJ (1985a) Organochlorine contaminants of wintering ducks foraging on Detroit River sediments. J Great Lakes Res, **11**(3): 231-246.

Smith AG, Francis JE, Dinsdale D, Manson MM, & Cabral JRP (1985b) Hepatocarcinogenicity of hexachlorobenzene in rats and the sex difference in hepatic iron status and development of porphyria. Carcinogenesis, **6**: 631-636.

Smith AG, Dinsdale D, Cabral JRP, & Wright AL (1987) Goitre and wasting induced in hamsters by hexachlorobenzene. Arch Toxicol, **60**: 343-349.

Smith AG, Cabral JRP, Carthew P, Francis JE, & Manson MM (1989) Carcinogenicity of iron in conjunction with a chlorinated environmental chemical, hexachlorobenzene, in C57BL/10ScSn mice. Int J Cancer, **43**: 492-496.

Smith AG, Francis JE, Green JA, Greig JB, Wolf CR, & Manson MM (1990) Sex-linked hepatic uroporphyria and the induction of cytochromes P450IA in rats caused by hexachlorobenzene and polyhalogenated biphenyls. Biochem Pharmacol, **40**: 2059-2068.

Smith AG, Carthew P, Francis JE, Cabral JRP, & Manson MM (1993) Enhancement by iron of hepatic neoplasia in rats caused by hexachlorobenzene. Carcinogenesis, **14**: 1381-1387.

Smith AG, Carthew P, Francis JE, & Ingebritsen K (1994) Influence of iron on the induction of hepatic tumors and porphyria by octachlorostyrene in C57BL/10ScSn mice. Cancer Lett, **81**: 145-150.

Solé M, Porte C, Pastor D, & Albaigés J (1994) Long-term trends of polychlorinated biphenyls and organochlorinated pesticides in mussels from the Western Mediterranean coast. Chemosphere, **28**(5): 897-903.

Somers JD, Goski BC, & Barrett MW (1987) Organochlorine residues in Northeastern Alberta otters. Bull Environ Contam Toxicol, **39**: 783-790.

Sopena de Kracoff YE, Ferramola de Sancovich AM, Sancovich HA, & Kleiman de Pisarev DL (1994) Effect of thyroidectomy and thyroxine on hexachlorobenzene induced porphyria. J Endocrinol Invest, **17**: 301-305.

Spigarelli JL, Going JE, & Li R (1986) Hexachlorobenzene levels in multimedia environmental samples from selected chemical production plants. In: Morris CR & Cabral JRP ed. Hexachlorobenzene: Proceedings of an International Symposium. Lyon, International Agency for Research on Cancer, pp 155-160 (IARC Scientific Publications No. 77).

Stacey CI, Perriman WS, & Whitney S (1985) Organochlorine pesticide residue levels in human milk: Western Australia, 1979-1980. Arch Environ Health, **40**(2): 102-108.

Stanley JS (1986) Broad scan analysis of the FY82 national human adipose tissue survey specimens - Volume I: Executive summary. Kansas City, Missouri, Midwest Research Institute (Prepared for the US Environmental Protection Agency, Office of Toxic Substances, Field Studies Branch) (EPA 560/5-86/035).

Stevens RJJ & Neilson MA (1989) Inter- and intralake distribution of trace contaminants in surface waters of the Great Lakes. J Great Lakes Res, **15**: 377-393.

Stevens MF, Ebell GF, & Psaila-Savona P (1993) Organochlorine pesticides in Western Australian nursing mothers. Med J Aust, **158**: 238-241.

Stewart FP & Smith AG (1987) Metabolism and covalent binding of hexachlorobenzene by isolated male and female rat hepatocytes. Biochem Pharmacol, **36**: 2232-2234.

Stewart FP, Manson MM, Cabral JRP, & Smith AG (1989) Hexachlorobenzene as a promoter of diethylnitrosamine-initiated hepatocarcinogenesis in rats and comparison with induction of porphyria. Carcinogenesis, **10**(7): 1225-1230.

Strik JJTWA (1986) Subacute toxicity of hexachlorobenzene. In: Morris CR & Cabral JRP ed. Hexachlorobenzene: Proceedings of an International Symposium. Lyon, International Agency for Research on Cancer, pp 335-342 (IARC Scientific Publications No. 77).

Stronkhorst J, Ysebaert TJ, Smedes F, Meininger PL, Dirksen S, & Boudewijn TJ (1993) Contaminants in eggs of some waterbird species from the Scheldt Estuary, SW Netherlands. Mar Pollut Bull, **26**(10): 572-578.

Sundlof SF, Hansen LG, Koritz GD, & Sundlof SM (1982) The pharmacokinetics of hexachlorobenzene in male beagles. Distribution, excretion and pharmacokinetic model. Drug Metab Dispos, **10**: 371-381.

Suns K, Craig GR, Crawford G, Rees GA, Tosine H, & Osborne J (1983) Organochlorine contaminant residues in spottail shiner (*Notropis hudsonius*) from the Niagara River. J Great Lakes Res, **9**: 335-340.

Suns K, Crawford GE, Russell DD, & Clement RE (1985) Temporal trends and spatial distribution of organochlorine and mercury residues in Great Lakes spottail shiners (1975-1983). Rexdale, Ontario, Ontario Ministry of the Environment, Water Resources Branch.

Swindoll CM & Applehans FM (1987) Factors influencing the accumulation of sediment-sorbed hexachlorobiphenyl by midge larvae. Bull Environ Contam Toxicol, **39**: 1055-1062.
Szymczyński GA, Waliszewski SM, Tuszewski M, & Pyda P (1986) Chlorinated pesticides levels in human adipose tissue in the district of Poznań. J Environ Sci Health, **A21**(1): 5-14.

Tanabe S, Subramanian AN, Ramesh A, Kumaran PL, Miyazaki N, & Tatsukawa R (1993) Persistent organochlorine residues in dolphins from the Bay of Bengal, South India. Mar Pollut Bull, **26**(6): 311-316.

Tehseen WM, Hansen LG, Wood SG, & Hanif M (1994) Assessment of chemical contaminants in water and sediment samples from Degh Nala in the province of Punjab, Pakistan. Arch Environ Contam Toxicol, **26**: 79-89.

Teschke R, Bolsen K, Landmann H, & Goerz G (1983) Effect of hexachlorobenzene on the activities of hepatic alcohol metabolizing enzymes. Biochem Pharmacol, **32**: 1745-1751.

Tetra Tech Inc. (1986) Development of sediment quality values for Puget Sound: Volume 1 (Prepared for Puget Sound Dredged Disposal Analysis and Puget Sound Estuary Program, Bellevue, Washington).

Theiss JC, Stoner GD, Shimkin MB, & Weisburger EK (1977) Test for carcinogenicity of organic contaminants of United States drinking waters by pulmonary tumor response in Strain A mice. Cancer Res, **37**: 2717-2720.

Thomas W, Simon H, & Rüling Å (1985) Classification of plant species by their organic (PAH, PCB, BHC) and inorganic (heavy metals) trace pollutant concentrations. Sci Total Environ, **46**: 83-94.

Thomson BA, Davidson WR, & Lovett AM (1980) Applications of a versatile technique for trace analysis: Atmospheric pressure negative chemical ionization. Environ Health Perspect, **36**: 77-84.

Tobin P (1986) Known and potential sources of hexachlorobenzene. In: Morris CR & Cabral JRP ed. Hexachlorobenzene: Proceedings of an International Symposium. Lyon, International Agency for Research on Cancer, pp 3-11 (IARC Scientific Publications No. 77).

To-Figueras J, Rodamilans M, Gómez-Catalán J, & Corbella J (1986) Hexachlorobenzene residues in the general population of Barcelona, Spain. In: Morris CR & Cabral JRP ed. Hexachlorobenzene: Proceedings of an International Symposium. Lyon, International Agency for Research on Cancer, p 147 (IARC Scientific Publications No. 77).

To-Figueras J, Gómez-Catalán J, Rodamilans M, & Corbella J (1992) Sulphur derivative of hexachlorobenzene in human urine. Hum Exp Toxicol, **11**: 271-273.

To-Figueras J, Barrot C, Rodamilans M, Gómez-Catalán J, Torra M, Brunet M, Sabater F, & Corbella J (1995) Accumulation of hexachlorobenzene in humans: a long standing risk. Hum Exp Toxicol, **14**: 20-23.

Topp E, Scheunert I, & Korte K (1989) Kinetics of the uptake of 14C-labelled chlorinated benzenes from soil by plants. Ecotoxicol Environ Saf, **17**: 157-166.

Trapp M, Baukloh V, Bohnet H-G, & Heeschen W (1984) Pollutants in human follicular fluid. Fertil Steril, **42**(1): 146-148.

US EPA (1980) Analysis of pesticide residues in human and environmental samples: A compilation of methods selected for use in pesticide monitoring programs. Research Triangle Park, North Carolina, US Environmental Protection Agency, Environmental Toxicology Division, Health Effects Research Laboratory (EPA 600/8-80-038).

US EPA (1982) Test methods: Methods of organic chemical analysis of municipal and industrial wastewater. Cincinnati, Ohio, US Environmental Protection Agency, Office of Research and Development, Environmental Monitoring and Support Laboratory (EPA 600/4-82-057).

US EPA (1985a) Health assessment document for chlorinated benzenes. Washington, DC, US Environmental Protection Agency, Office of Health and Environmental Assessment (EPA 600/8-84-015F).

US EPA (1985b) Drinking water criteria document for hexachlorobenzene. Cincinnati, Ohio, US Environmental Protection Agency, Environmental Criteria and Assessment Office (EPA 600/X-84-179-1).

US EPA (1986a) Exposure assessment for hexachlorobenzene. Washington, DC, US Environmental Protection Agency, Office of Pesticides and Toxic Substances (EPA 560/5-86-0(19).

US EPA (1986b) Test methods for evaluating solid waste, 3rd ed. Washington, DC, US Environmental Protection Agency, Office of Solid Waste and Emergency Response (SW 846).

US EPA (1988) Ambient aquatic life water quality criteria for hexachlorobenzene. Duluth, Minnesota, US Environmental Protection Agency, Office of Research and Development.

US FDA (US Food and Drug Administration) (1990) Residues in foods - 1988. J Assoc Off Anal Chem, **73**: 133A-152A.

US FDA (US Food and Drug Administration) (1991) Residues in foods - 1989. J Assoc Off Anal Chem, **74**: 127A-146A.

US FDA (US Food and Drug Administration) (1992) Residues in foods - 1990. J Assoc Off Anal Chem, **75**: 121A-141A.

Üstünbas HB, Öztürk MA, Hasanoglu E, & Dogan M (1994) Organochlorine pesticide residues in human milk in Kayseri. Hum Exp Toxicol, **13**: 299-302.

Van der Ven K, Van der Ven H, Thibold A, Bauer O, Kaisi M, Mbura J, Mhaya HN, Wever N, Diedrich K, & Krebs D (1992) Chorinated hydrocarbon content of fetal and maternal body tissues and fluids in full term pregnant women: a comparison of Germany versus Tanzania. Hum Reprod, **7**(1): 95-100.

Van Leeuwen CJ, Van der Zandt PTJ, Aldenberg T, Verhaar HJM, & Hermans JLM (1992) Application of QSARs, extrapolation and equilibrium partitioning in aquatic effects assessment: I. Narcotic industrial pollutants. Environ Toxicol Chem, **11**: 267-282.

Van Loveren H, Kranjc EI, Rombout PJA, Blommaert FA, & Vos JG (1990) Effects of ozone, hexachlorobenzene, and bis(tri-*n*-butyltin)oxide on natural killer activity in the rat lung. Toxicol Appl Pharmacol, **102**: 21-33.

Van Ommen B, Hendriks W, Bessems JGM, Geesink G, Müller F, & Van Bladeren PJ (1989) The relation between the oxidative biotransformation of hexachlorobenzene and its porphyrinogenic activity. Toxicol Appl Pharmacol, **100**: 517-528.

Van Raaij JAGM, Van den Berg KJ, & Notten WRF (1991a) Hexachlorobenzene and its metabolites pentachlorophenol and tetrachlorohydroquinone: interaction with thyroxine binding sites of rat thyroid hormone carriers *ex vivo* and *in vitro*. Toxicol Lett, **59**: 101-107.

Van Raaij JAGM, Van den Berg KJ, Engel R, Bragt PC, & Notten WRF (1991b) Effects of hexachlorobenzene and its metabolites pentachlorophenol and tetrachlorohydroquinone on serum thyroid hormone levels in rats. Toxicology, **67**: 107-116.

Van Raaij JAGM, Frijters CMG, & Van den Berg KJ (1993a) Hexachlorobenzene-induced hypothyroidism: involvement of different mechanisms by parent compound and metabolite. Biochem Pharmacol, **46**: 1385-1391.

Van Raaij JAGM, Kaptein E, Visser TJ, & Van den Berg KJ (1993b) Increased glucoronidation of thyroid hormone in hexachlorobenzene-treated rats. Biochem Pharmacol, **45**: 627-631.

Vaz R, Slorach SA, & Hofvander Y (1993) Organochlorine contaminants in Swedish human milk: studies conducted at the National Food Administration 1981-1990. Food Addit Contam, **10**(4): 407-418.

Villanueva EC, Jennings RW, Burse VW, & Kimbrough RD (1974) Evidence of chlorodibenzo-p-dioxin and chlorodibenzofuran in hexachlorobenzene. J Agric Food Chem, **22**: 916-917.

Villeneuve DC, Panopio LG, & Grant DL (1974) Placental transfer of hexachlorobenzene in the rabbit. Environ Physiol Biochem, **4**: 112-115.

Vincent SH, Smith AG, & Muller-Eberhard U (1989) Modulation of hepatic heme-binding Z protein in mice by the porphyrogenic carcinogens griseofulvin and hexachlorobenzene. Cancer Lett, **45**: 109-114.

Vos JG (1986) Immunotoxicity of hexachlorobenzene. In: Morris CR & Cabral JRP ed. Hexachlorobenzene: Proceedings of an International Symposium. Lyon, International Agency for Research on Cancer, pp 347-356 (IARC Scientific Publications No. 77).

Vos JG, Breeman HA, & Benschop H (1968) The occurrence of the fungicide hexachlorobenzene in wild birds and its toxicological importance: a preliminary communication. Meded Fac. Landbouwwet Rijksuniv Gent, **33**: 1263-1269.

Vos JG, Van der Maas HL Musch A, & Ram E (1971) Toxicity of hexachlorobenzene in Japanese quail with special reference to porphyria, liver damage, reproduction and tissue residues. Toxicol Appl Pharmacol, **18**: 944-957.

Vos JG, Botterweg PF, Strik JJTWA, & Koeman JH (1972) Experimental studies with HCB in birds. TNO-Nieuws, **27**: 599-603.

Vos JG, Van Logten MJ, Kreeftenberg JG, & Kruizinga W (1979a) Hexachlorobenzene-induced stimulation of the humoral immune response in rats. Ann NY Acad Sci, **320**: 535-550.

Vos JG, Van Logten MJ, Kreeftenberg JG, Steerenberg PA, & Kruizinga W (1979b) Effect of hexachlorobenzene on the immune system of rats following combined pre- and postnatal exposure. Drug Chem Toxicol, **2**: 61-76.

Vos JG, Brouwer GMJ, Van Leeuwen FXR, & Wagenaar SJ (1983) Toxicity of hexachlorobenzene in the rat following combined pre- and post-natal exposure: comparison of effects on the immune system, liver and lung. In: Parke DV, Gibson GG, & Hubbard R ed. Immunotoxicology. New York, London, Academic Press, pp 219-235.

Vos RME, Snoek MC, Van Berkel WJH, Müller F, & Van Bladeren PJ (1988) Differential induction of rat hepatic glutathione S-transferase isoenzymes by hexachlorobenzene and benzyl isothiocyanate: comparison with induction by phenobarbital and 3-methylcholanthrene. Biochem Pharmacol, **37**: 1077-1082.

Wada O, Yano Y, Urata G, & Nakao K (1968) Behavior of hepatic microsomal cytochromes after treatment of mice with drugs known to disturb porphyrin metabolism in liver. Biochem Pharmacol, **17**: 595-603.

Wang M-J & Jones KC (1994) Occurrence of chlorobenzenes in nine United Kingdom retail vegetables. J Agric Food Chem, **42**: 2322-2328.

Washington State Department of Ecology (1990) Proposed sediment management standards rule (September 18, 1990). Washington State Register, issue 90-19.

Watts RR, Hodgson DW, Christ HL, & Moseman RF (1980) Improved method for hexachlorobenzene and mirex determination with hexachlorobenzene confirmation in adipose tissue: Collaborative study. J Assoc Off Anal Chem, **63**(5): 1128-1134.

Weisenberg E, Arad I, Grauer F, & Sahm Z (1985) Polychlorinated biphenyls and organochlorine insecticides in human milk in Israel. Arch Environ Contam Toxicol, **14**: 517-521.

Wells DE, Campbell LA, Ross HM, Thompson PM, & Lockyer CH (1994) Organochlorine residues in harbour porpoise and bottlenose dolphins stranded on the coast of Scotland, 1988-1991. Sci Total Environ, **151**: 77-99.

WHO (1993) Guidelines for drinking-water quality - Volume 1: Recommendations, 2nd ed. Geneva, World Health Organization, p 84.

Wickström K, Pyysalo H, & Siimes MA (1983) Levels of chlordane, hexachlorobenzene, PCB and DDT compounds in Finnish human milk in 1982. Bull Environ Contam Toxicol, **31**: 251-256.

Williams DT, Lebel GL, & Junkins E (1984) A comparison of organochlorine residues in human adipose tissue autopsy samples from two Ontario municipalities. J Toxicol Environ Health, **13**: 19-29.

Williams DT, Lebel GL, & Junkins E (1988) Organohalogen residues in human adipose autopsy samples from six Ontario municipalities. J Assoc Off Anal Chem, **71**: 410-414.

Wilson DM & Wan MTK (1982) Hexachlorobenzene: Industrial and agricultural sources in British Columbia. Vancouer, Environment Canada, Environmental Protection Service (Regional Program Report No. 82-07).

Witte H, Langenohl T, & Offenbacher SAG (1988a) Investigation of the entry of organic pollutants into soils and plants through the use of sewage sludge in agriculture. Part A: Organic pollutant load in sewage sludge. Korresp Abwasser, **13**: 118-125.

Witte H, Langenohl T, & Offenbacher SAG (1988b) Investigation of the entry of organic pollutants into soils and plants through the use of sewage sludge in agriculture. Part B: Impact of the application of sewage sludge on organic matter content in soil and plants. Korresp Abwasser, **13**: 126-136.

Yamaguchi Y, Kawano M, & Tatsukawa R (1986) Tissue distribution and excretion of hexabromobenzene (HBB) and hexachlorobenzene (HCB) administered to rats. Chemosphere, **15**: 453-459.

Yang RSH, Pittman KA, Rourke DR, & Stein VB (1978) Pharmacokinetics and metabolism of hexachlorobenzene in the rat and the rhesus monkey. J Agric Food Chem, **26**: 1076-1083.

RÉSUMÉ ET CONCLUSIONS

1. Identité, propriétés chimiques et physiques et méthodes d'analyse

L'hexachlorobenzène (HCB) est un composé organique chloré modérément volatil. Il est pratiquement insoluble dans l'eau, mais extrêmement soluble dans les lipides et présente une tendance à la bioaccumulation. L'hexachlorobenzène de qualité technique contient jusqu'à 2% d'impuretés, dont la principale est le pentachlorobenzène. Les autres consistent en dibenzo-*p*-dioxines, dibenzofuranes et biphényles fortement substitués par le chlore. L'analyse des échantillons biologiques ou prélevés dans l'environnement comporte généralement une extraction préliminaire de la prise d'essai, souvent suivie d'une purification, après quoi les extraits organiques sont soumis soit à une chromatographie en phase gazeuse couplée à la spectrométrie de masse (GC/MS), soit à une chromatographie en phase gazeuse avec détection par capture d'électrons (GC/ECD).

2. Sources d'exposition humaine et environnementale

L'hexachlorobenzène a été utilisé un temps comme fongicide pour traiter les semences, mais il n'est plus actuellement utilisé à cet effet dans la plupart des pays. Il continue néanmoins à être libéré dans l'environnement à partir d'un certain nombre de sources, notamment lors de l'épandage de pesticides organochlorés, ou encore lorsque les sous-produits de la préparation des solvants, composés aromatiques ou pesticides chlorés sont rejetés sans précautions, incomplètement brûlés ou s'échappent de décharges anciennes.

3. Transport, distribution et transformation dans l'environnement

L'hexachlorobenzène est réparti dans tout l'environnement du fait de sa mobilité et de sa persistance, même s'il se décompose lentement dans l'air sous l'action de la lumière et dans le sol sous l'action des microorganismes. Dans la troposphère, il est transporté sur de grandes distances et s'élimine de l'air en se déposant sur le sol et sur l'eau. On a fait état d'une bioamplification notable le long de la chaîne alimentaire.

4. Concentrations dans l'environnement et exposition humaine

Un peu partout dans le monde, l'hexachlorobenzène est présent, à distance de ses sources, sous faible concentration dans l'air ambiant (quelques ng/m^3 ou moins) ainsi que dans l'eau de boisson et les eaux de surface (quelques ng/litre tout au plus). Cependant, au voisinage des points d'émission, on a pu mesurer des concentrations plus élevées. Ce composé s'accumule dans les milieux biologiques et on en a décelé la présence chez des invertébrés, des poissons, des reptiles, des oiseaux et des mammifères (y compris l'Homme) à distance des points d'émission, en particulier dans les tissus adipeux des organismes situés aux niveaux trophiques supérieurs. Chez la population humaine de divers pays, on en a mesuré dans les tissus adipeux des quantités qui vont, en moyenne, de quelques dizaines à quelques centaines de ng/g de poids humide. En se fondant sur les quantités représentatives d'hexachlorobenzène présentes dans l'air, l'eau et les denrées alimentaires, on peut estimer à une valeur comprise entre 0,0004 et 0,003 µg/kg de poids corporel, la dose absorbée journalièrement par un adulte de la population générale. Cet apport se fait principalement par la voie alimentaire. Du fait de la présence d'hexachlorobenzène dans le lait maternel, on estime que dans les différents pays les enfants nourris au sein en reçoivent quotidiennement une quantité comprise entre $< 0,018$ et 5,1 µg/kg de poids corporel. Les études consacrées à l'évolution de la quantité d'hexachlorobenzène présente dans l'organisme humain montrent, pour la plupart, que l'exposition de la population générale a baissé dans de nombreux endroits, entre les années 70 et le milieu de la décennie actuelle.

5. Cinétique et métabolisme chez l'Homme et les animaux de laboratoire

On manque de données toxicocinétiques chez l'Homme. L'hexachlorobenzène est facilement résorbé par la voie orale chez l'animal d'expérience, mais il franchit mal la barrière cutanée (on ne possède pas de données concernant l'inhalation). Chez l'Homme et l'animal, il s'accumule dans les tissus riches en lipides, comme les tissus adipeux, le cortex surrénalien, la moelle osseuse, la peau et certains tissus endocriniens. En outre, il peut être transmis à la progéniture par l'intermédiaire du lait maternel ou en traversant la barrière placentaire. La métabolisation de l'hexachlorobenzène est limitée et ses principaux métabolites urinaires sont le pentachlorophénol, la tétrachlorhydroquinone et le pentachlorothiophénol. La demi-vie d'élimination de l'hexachlorobenzène va d'environ un mois chez les rats et les lapins à 2 ou 3 ans chez le singe.

6. Effets sur les animaux de laboratoire et dans les épreuves *in vitro*

L'hexachlorobenzène présente une faible toxicité aiguë pour les animaux de laboratoire (1000 à 10 000 mg/kg de poids corporel). L'expérimentation animale montre en outre que ce composé n'est pas irritant pour la peau ou les yeux et ne provoque pas de sensibilisation chez le cobaye.

Les données dont on dispose au sujet de la toxicité générale de l'hexachlorobenzène indiquent que celle-ci s'exerce notamment au niveau de la voie de biosynthèse de l'hème. Chez plusieurs espèces de mammifères de laboratoire exposés à de l'hexachlorobenzène, on a constaté une élévation des concentrations de porphyrines ou de leurs précurseurs dans les excréta ainsi que dans divers tissus, notamment le tissu hépatique. De nombreuses études ont relevé des cas de porphyrie chez des rats exposés de manière chronique ou subchronique à de l'hexachlorobenzène administré par voie orale à des doses quotidiennes comprises entre 2,5 et 15 mg par kg de poids corporel. Chez des porcs à qui on faisait ingérer ce composé en doses quotidiennes égales ou supérieures à 0,5 mg par kg de poids corporel, on a observé une augmentation de l'excrétion des coproporphyrines (aucun effet n'a été observé dans cette étude à la dose de 0,05 mg/kg). On a également montré que l'exposition à l'hexachlorobenzène affectait de nombreux organes ou systèmes (comme le foie, les poumons, les reins, la thyroïde, la peau ainsi que le système nerveux et le système immunitaire) mais ces effets n'ont pas été aussi souvent signalés que la porphyrie.

L'hexachlorobenzène est un inducteur du cytochrome P-450 de type mixte. Il possède des propriétés phénobarbital-inductibles et 3-méthylcholantrène-inductibles. Il se fixe sur le récepteur Ah.

Lors d'études longitudinales sur des rats, on a observé à plusieurs reprises des effets bénins (modifications histopathologiques, induction d'enzymes) chez les animaux recevant des doses quotidiennes comprises entre 0,25 et 0,6 mg de composé par kg de poids corporel. La dose sans effet observable obtenue dans ces études se situait entre 0,05 et 0,07 mg d'hexachlorobenzène par kg de poids corporel et par jour. Chez des visons femelles, on a observé une modification de la concentration de neurotransmetteurs dans l'hypothalamus après administration prolongée du composé par la voie alimentaire à la dose quotidienne de 0,16 mg par kg de poids corporel. Les mêmes constatations ont été faites dans la progéniture de ces animaux, qui avait été exposée pendant les périodes gestationnelle et périnatale. Lors d'études subchroniques sur des rats on a constaté une modification de l'homéostase calcique et des paramètres ostéomorphométriques à la dose quotidienne de 0,7 mg/kg de poids corporel, mais pas à celle de 0,07 mg/kg.

Un certain nombre d'études *in vivo* ont été effectuées sur des rongeurs afin de mettre en évidence la cancérogénicité éventuelle de l'hexachlorobenzène. Chez des hamsters qui avaient reçu une nourriture contenant de l'hexachlorobenzène à la dose moyenne de 4, 8 ou 16 mg/kg de poids corporel, on a observé chez les deux sexes et à toutes les doses un accroissement de l'incidence des carcinomes hépatocellulaires. Aux doses de 8 et 16 mg/kg, on constatait la présence d'hémangioendothéliomes et à la dose la plus forte, d'adénomes de la thyroïde chez les mâles. En exposant pendant 120 semaines des souris à ce composé par la voie alimentaire aux doses quotidiennes respectives de 6, 12 et 24 mg/kg de poids corporel, on a provoqué un accroissement de l'incidence des carcinomes hépatocellulaires chez les deux sexes aux deux doses les plus élevées, mais cet accroissement n'était pas significatif, sauf chez les femelles exposées à la dose la plus forte. *In utero,* l'exposition de rats par la voie orale ou lactationnelle à des doses alimentaires quotidiennes d'hexachlorobenzène allant de 0,01 à 1,5 mg/kg de poids corporel (mâles) ou de 1,9 mg/kg (femelles) pendant des périodes pouvant durer jusqu'à 130 semaines *post utero*, c'est-à-dire la durée de vie moyenne, a entraîné à la dose la plus forte un accroissement de l'incidence des nodules hépatiques néoplasiques et des phéochromocytomes surrénaliens chez les femelles et un excès d'adénomes parathyroïdiens chez les mâles. Lors d'une autre étude chronique effectuée sur des rats, on a exposé les animaux, par la voie alimentaire et pendant des durées allant jusqu'à 2 ans, à des doses journalières moyennes de 4-5 et 8-9 mg/kg de poids corporel. Les effets constatés consistaient en une augmentation de l'incidence des hépatomes et des adénomes rénaux aux deux doses et chez les deux sexes. Chez les femelles, on observait en outre une augmentation de l'incidence des carcinomes hépatocellulaires, des adénomes et des carcinomes des voies biliaires, des phéochromocytomes et des adénomes du cortex surrénalien. On a également signalé une incidence élevée des tumeurs du foie dans un certain nombre d'études plus limitées au cours desquelles on avait administré une seule dose d'hexachlorobenzène par la voie alimentaire à de petits groupes de rates. Par ailleurs, on a observé qu'après exposition subchronique par voie alimentaire à ce composé, des souris, des hamsters et des rats avaient présenté des tumeurs du foie, des voies biliaires, du rein, du thymus, de la rate et des ganglions lymphatiques. Le même type d'exposition favorise l'apparition de tumeurs hépatiques chez des souris sous l'action de terphényles polychlorés et chez des rats, sous l'action de la diéthylnitrosamine.

Sauf dans le cas des tumeurs rénales chez les rats mâles (qui, du moins en partie, semblent résulter d'une dégénérescence hyaline) et des hépatomes chez les rats des deux sexes (qui pourraient résulter de réactions hyperplasiques à la nécrose hépatocellulaire), on n'a pas pu trouver d'études mécanistiques concernant les divers types de tumeurs provoquées par l'hexachlorobenzène et le risque encouru à cet égard par l'Homme.

L'hexachlorobenzène n'a guère d'aptitude à provoquer directement des mutations géniques, des lésions chromosomiques ou la réparation de l'ADN. Il s'est révélé faiblement mutagène lors de quelques-unes des études portant sur des bactéries et des levures, mais il convient de noter que chacune de ces études comportait des limitations. Il y a également des signes d'un faible taux de liaison à l'ADN *in vitro* et *in vivo*, mais dans une proportion très inférieure à celle que l'on attendrait d'une substance cancérogène génotoxique.

Lors d'études sur la reproduction, des doses d'hexachlorobenzène ne dépassant pas 0,1 mg par kg de poids corporel qu'on avait fait ingérer quotidiennement pendant 90 jours à des singes, ont provoqué des anomalies dans la structure microscopique et l'ultrastructure de l'épithélium germinatif superficiel, structures qui constituent une cible inhabituelle pour des toxines ovariennes. Cette dose a également endommagé l'ultrastructure des cellules germinales primordiales. Alors même que ces sites étaient spécifiquement attaqués et présentaient des lésions d'autant plus importantes que la dose était plus forte, le développement folliculaire, ovocytaire et embryonnaire restait normal, ce qui semble indiquer que l'hexachlorobenzène a un site d'action à localisation spécifiquement ovarienne. Chez les mâles, la fonction de reproduction n'est affectée qu'à des doses beaucoup plus élevées (entre 30 et 221 mg/kg p.c. par jour), comme l'ont montré un certain nombre d'études effectuées sur plusieurs espèces n'appartenant pas à l'ordre des primates.

Des rats et des chats exposés par la voie transplacentaire ou lactationnelle à des doses quotidiennes d'hexachlorobenzène comprises entre 3 et 4 mg/kg p.c. ont présenté des signes d'hépatotoxicité et on a également constaté des effets délétères sur la survie et la croissance de leur progéniture. Dans certains cas, il y avait à ces doses - ou à des doses plus élevées - une réduction de l'effectif des portées et un nombre accru de mortinaissances. (En général, les ratons et les chatons à la mamelle étaient plus souvent affectés - et à des doses plus faibles - que les embryons et les foetus). Chez la progéniture de visons qui recevaient une alimentation ne contenant pas plus de 1 mg d'hexachlorobenzène par kg de nourriture (soit environ 0,16 mg/kg p.c. par jour), on a constaté une réduction du poids de naissance et un accroissement de la mortalité au sevrage. Quelques études ont mis en évidence des anomalies squelettiques ou rénales chez les foetus de rats et de souris exposés à de l'hexachlorobenzène pendant la gestation, mais les doses qui produisaient ces anomalies n'étaient pas toxiques pour les mères. Par ailleurs, le lien de ces anomalies avec la prise d'hexachlorobenzène n'a pas été formellement établi. Dans deux études, dont l'une comportait une exposition transplacentaire et postnatale, on a observé des anomalies du développement neurocomportemental des ratons après exposition *in utero*, les mères ayant reçu par voie orale des doses quotidiennes d'hexachlorobenzène allant de 0,64 à 2,5 mg/kg de poids corporel.

Selon un certain nombre d'études, l'hexachlorobenzène aurait des effets délétères sur le système immunitaire. Chez des rats et des singes exposés à des doses quotidiennes comprises entre 3 et 120 mg d'hexachlorobenzène par kg de poids corporel, on a constaté des modifications histopathologiques au niveau du thymus, de la rate, des ganglions lymphatiques et des tissus lymphoïdes pulmonaires. Chez des chiens beagle exposés de façon chronique à des doses quotidiennes correspondant à 0,12 mg de composé par kg p.c., on a observé une hyperplasie nodulaire du tissu lymphoïde gastrique. Un certain nombre d'études menées sur des rats ont montré qu'après plusieurs semaines d'exposition à de l'hexachlorobenzène par la voie alimentaire, il y avait stimulation de l'immunité humorale, et dans une moindre mesure, de l'immunité à médiation cellulaire, sans modification de la fonction des macrophages. A des doses quotidiennes ne dépassant pas 4 mg de composé par kg de nourriture (environ 0,2 mg par kg p.c.), administrées pendant la gestation, pendant le maternage et jusqu'à l'âge de 5 semaines, il y a eu augmentation de la réponse immunitaire à médiation cellulaire et de la réponse immunitaire humorale ainsi qu'une accumulation de macrophages dans le tissu pulmonaire des ratons. Par contre, la plupart des études effectuées sur des souris ont fait ressortir les propriétés immunosuppressives de l'hexachlorobenzène; des doses ne dépassant pas 0,5 à 0,6 mg/kg de poids corporel administrées quotidiennement pendant plusieurs semaines ont eu les effets suivants: diminution de la résistance à une infection leishmanienne ou à une épreuve cancérogène par exposition à des cellules tumorales, réduction de l'activité cytotoxique des macrophages spléniques et de l'hypersensibilité retardée chez la progéniture après exposition *in utero* ou pendant la période de maternage. Lors d'un certain nombre d'études portant sur diverses souches de rats, on a constaté qu'une exposition de brève durée ou une exposition subchronique à de l'hexachlorobenzène modifiait la fonction thyroïdienne, comme on pouvait en juger d'après la réduction de la thyroxine sérique libre ou totale (T_4) et souvent, mais dans une moindre mesure, de la triiodothyronine (T_3).

7. Effets sur l'Homme

La plupart des données que l'on possède au sujet des effets de l'hexachlorobenzène sur l'Homme, proviennent d'intoxications accidentelles qui se sont produites en Turquie en 1955-59, avec plus de 600 cas répertoriés de porphyrie cutanée tardive. Lors de cet accident, on a observé des troubles du métabolisme des porphyrines, des lésions cutanées, des hyperpigmentations, des hypertrichoses, des hépatomégalies, des hypertrophies de la thyroïde et des ganglions lymphatiques, avec, dans environ la moitié des cas, une ostéoporose et une arthrite, principalement d'ailleurs, chez les enfants. Les enfants nourris au sein dont la mère avait été exposée, présentaient des lésions appelées *pembe yara*, c'est-à-dire "lésions roses", et la plupart d'entre eux sont décédés dans l'année. On dispose de quelques données concernant des cas de porphyrie cutanée tardive chez des personnes ayant subi une exposition relativement intense à l'hexachlorobenzène sur leur lieu de travail ou dans leur environnement général.

Les quelques études épidémiologiques disponibles concernant le cancer souffrent d'un certain nombre d'insuffisances: effectif réduit, exposition à l'hexachlorobenzène mal caractérisée ou exposition simultanée à de nombreux autres agents, et ne permettent pas d'évaluer la cancérogénicité de ce composé pour l'Homme.

8. Effets sur les autres êtres vivants au laboratoire et dans leur milieu naturel

Lors d'études sur la toxicité aiguë de l'hexachlorobenzène pour les organismes aquatiques, on a constaté que l'exposition à des concentrations de l'ordre de 1 à 17 µg/litre réduisait la production de chlorophylle chez les algues ainsi que la reproduction chez les ciliés, et qu'en outre, elle provoquait la mort des crevettes roses et des crevettes américaines du genre *Hippolyte*, mais elle n'a pas provoqué la mort de poissons d'eau douce ou de mer. Lors d'études à plus long terme, on a constaté que la croissance de certaines algues et protozoaires dulçaquicoles sensibles étaient affectée à une concentration d'hexachlorobenzène de 1 µg/litre et que des concentrations d'environ 3 µg/litre provoquaient la mort d'amphipodes et de perches appartenant à l'espèce *Micropterus salmoides*.

9. Evaluation des risques pour la santé humaine et des effets sur l'environnement

9.1 Effets sur la santé

Le Groupe de travail a conclu que les données disponibles sont suffisantes pour que l'on puisse formuler des valeurs-guides relatives aux effets cancérogènes et non cancérogènes de l'hexachlorobenzène.

En ce qui concerne les effets non cancérogènes constatés sur le foie à dose élevée chez des porcs et des rats exposés par la voie orale et en se basant sur la dose sans effet observable la plus faible (0,05 mg/kg de poids corporel par jour), on arrive, compte tenu d'un facteur d'incertitude de 300 (10x pour les variations interspécifiques, 10x pour les variations intraspécifiques et 3x pour la gravité de l'effet), à une TDI de 0,17 µg/kg de poids corporel.

La méthode utilisée pour déterminer la valeur-guide relative aux effets cancérogènes repose sur la dose tumorigène TD_5, c'est-à-dire la dose ingérée qui provoque une augmentation de 5% de l'incidence tumorale chez les animaux de laboratoire. D'après les résultats d'une étude de cancérogénicité portant sur deux générations de rats et en faisant appel à un modèle multiphasique, on obtient une TD_5 de 0,81 mg/kg de poids corporel par jour, l'effet retenu étant la formation de nodules cancéreux hépatiques chez les femelles. Compte tenu de l'insuffisance des données mécanistiques, on a appliqué un facteur d'incertitude de 5000 pour calculer la valeur-guide chiffrée à 0,16 µg/kg de poids corporel par jour.

9.2 Effets sur l'environnement

Le Groupe de travail a remarqué qu'il existe très peu d'études expérimentales à partir desquelles on puisse procéder à une évaluation du risque écologique. La concentration d'hexachlorobenzène dans les eaux de surface est généralement inférieure de plusieurs ordres de grandeur à celle qui pourrait être dangereuse pour les organismes aquatiques, sauf dans certains endroits fortement pollués. Toutefois, les concentrations d'hexachlorobenzène relevées dans les oeufs d'oiseaux de mer et de rapaces en différents lieux du globe sont proches de celles qui provoquent une diminution du poids des embryons chez la mouette argentée (1500 µg/kg), ce qui incite à penser que le composé pourrait être embryotoxique pour certaines espèces sensibles d'oiseaux. De même, les concentrations d'hexachlorobenzène dans les poissons de divers endroits du monde sont du même ordre de grandeur que la dose de 1000 µg/kg qui entraîne une réduction du poids de naissance et une augmentation de la mortalité chez la progéniture de visons. Cela incite à penser que ce composé pourrait avoir des effets indésirables chez les visons et éventuellement chez d'autres mammifères piscivores.

10. Conclusions

a) L'hexachlorobenzène est un composé chimique persistant qui subit une bioaccumulation du fait de sa liposolubilité et de sa résistance à la décomposition.

b) L'expérimentation animale montre que l'hexachlorobenzène provoque des cancers et affecte de nombreux organes, tissus et systèmes comme le foie, les poumons, les reins, la thyroïde, les tissus des gonades, le système nerveux et le système immunitaire.

c) En ce qui concerne l'Homme, on a pu observer, à l'occasion d'une forte exposition d'origine accidentelle, les manifestations cliniques d'une intoxication par l'hexachlorobenzène qui se traduisaient par une porphyrie cutanée tardive chez les enfants et les adultes et par la mort chez des nourrissons alimentés au sein.

d) Il est justifié de prendre diverses mesures pour réduire la quantité d'hexachlorobenzène présente dans l'environnement.

e) On a proposé les valeurs-guides à visée sanitaire suivantes pour la dose totale ingérée quotidiennement (TDI): en ce qui concerne les effets non cancérogènes, 0,17 µg/kg de poids corporel par jour ; en ce qui concerne les effets cancérogènes, 0,16 µg/kg de poids corporel par jour.

1. RÉSUMEN Y CONCLUSIONES

1. Identidad, propiedades físicas y químicas y métodos analíticos

El hexaclorobenceno (HCB) es un compuesto orgánico clorado de volatilidad moderada. Es prácticamente insoluble en el agua, pero es muy liposoluble y bioacumulativo. El HCB de calidad técnica contiene hasta un 2% de impurezas, en su mayor parte pentaclorobenceno; el resto incluye dibenzo-*p*-dioxinas, dibenzofuranos y bifenilos altamente clorados. Para determinar el HCB en el medio ambiente y en material biológico se procede por lo general a extraer la muestra mediante disolventes orgánicos, a lo que sigue con frecuencia un paso de limpieza, a fin de obtener extractos orgánicos analizables mediante cromatografía de gases/espectrometría de masas (GC/MS) o cromatografía de gases con detección de captura de electrones (GC/ECD).

2. Fuentes de exposición humana y ambiental

Hubo un tiempo en que el HCB se utilizó mucho en la limpieza de semillas para prevenir las enfermedades micóticas de los cereales, pero ese uso se abandonó en la mayor parte de los países en los años setenta. El HCB se sigue liberando en el medio ambiente a partir de diversas fuentes, que incluyen el uso de algunos plaguicidas clorados, procesos de combustión incompleta y viejos vertederos, así como los métodos inapropiados de producción y de eliminación de desechos en la fabricación de disolventes clorados, compuestos aromáticos clorados y plaguicidas clorados.

3. Transporte, distribución y transformación en el medio ambiente

El HCB se distribuye por todo el medio ambiente porque es móvil y persistente, aunque se produce una lenta fotodegradación en el aire y una degradación microbiana en el suelo. En la troposfera el HCB es transportado a grandes distancias y es eliminado de la fase aérea por su depósito en el agua y el suelo. Se ha informado de que se produce una importante bioamplificación del HCB a través de la cadena trófica.

4. Niveles ambientales y exposición humana

Se encuentran concentraciones bajas de HCB en el aire ambiental (a lo sumo unos pocos ng/m^3), en el agua de bebida y en las aguas superficiales (a lo sumo unos pocos ng/litro) de zonas alejadas del punto emisor en todo el mundo. No obstante, se han hallado concentraciones más altas cerca de los puntos emisores. El HCB es bioacumulativo y se ha detectado en invertebrados, peces, reptiles, aves y mamíferos (incluido el hombre) lejos de los puntos emisores, particularmente en el tejido adiposo de organismos de los niveles tróficos más altos. Los niveles medios en el tejido adiposo de la población humana general en diversos países van de decenas a centenas de ng/g de peso en fresco. Considerando los niveles representativos de HCB en el aire, el agua y los alimentos, se estima que la ingesta total de HCB por los adultos de la población general está comprendida entre 0,0004 y 0,003 µg/kg de peso corporal al día. Esa ingesta se realiza principalmente a través de los alimentos. Debido a la presencia de HCB en la leche materna, se ha estimado que la ingesta media por los lactantes alimentados al pecho en diversos países va de < 0,018 a 5,1 µg/kg de peso corporal al día. Los resultados de la mayoría de los estudios realizados acerca de las concentraciones de HCB en los alimentos y en los tejidos humanos a lo largo del tiempo indican que la exposición de la población general al HCB disminuyó desde los años setenta hasta mediados de los noventa en muchos lugares. Sin embargo, esa tendencia no se ha confirmado con claridad durante el último decenio en otros lugares.

5. Cinética y metabolismo en animales de laboratorio y en el ser humano

No hay suficientes datos sobre la toxicocinética en el hombre. El HCB es absorbido rápidamente por vía oral por los animales de experimentación, y escasamente a través de la piel (no existen datos sobre la inhalación). En los animales y en los seres humanos, el HCB se acumula en los tejidos ricos en lípidos, como el tejido adiposo, la corteza suprarrenal, la médula ósea, la piel y algunos tejidos endocrinos, y puede transmitirse a la descendencia a través tanto de la placenta como de la leche materna. El HCB sufre un metabolismo limitado, generando pentaclorofenol, tetraclorohidroquinona y pentaclorotiofenol como principales metabolitos en la orina. Las semividas de eliminación del HCB están comprendidas entre aproximadamente un mes en la rata y el conejo y 2 ó 3 años en el mono.

6. Efectos en animales de laboratorio y en las pruebas *in vitro*

La toxicidad aguda del HCB en los animales de experimentación es baja (1000 x 10 000 mg/kg de peso corporal). En los estudios con animales, el HCB no causa irritación cutánea ni ocular y no tiene efectos de sensibilización en el cobayo.

Los datos disponibles acerca de la toxicidad sistémica del HCB indican que las vías de la biosíntesis del grupo hemo son una importante diana de la toxicidad del hexaclorobenceno. Se han hallado niveles elevados de porfirinas o de precursores de la porfirina, o de ambas cosas, en el hígado, en otros tejidos y en las excretas de varias especies de mamíferos de laboratorio expuestos al HCB. Se ha informado de la aparición de porfiria en varios estudios realizados con ratas expuestas por vía oral crónica o subcrónica a dosis entre 2,5 y 15 mg de HCB/kg de peso corporal al día. La excreción de coproporfirinas aumentó en cerdos que ingirieron 0,5 mg de HCB/kg de peso corporal al día o más (en el último estudio no se observó ningún efecto con 0,05 mg de HCB/kg de peso corporal al día). Se ha visto también que la exposición repetida al HCB afecta a una amplia gama de sistemas orgánicos (entre ellos el hígado, los pulmones, los riñones, la tiroides, la piel y los sistemas nervioso e inmunitario), aunque las referencias a estos efectos son menos frecuentes que las relacionadas con la porfiria.

El HCB es un inductor de tipo mixto del citocromo P-450, con propiedades inducibles por el fenobarbital y por el 3-metilcolantreno. Se sabe que se une al receptor Ah.

Por lo que se refiere a los estudios crónicos, en ratas expuestas a dosis de 0,25 a 0,6 mg de HCB/kg peso corporal al día se observaron efectos leves en el hígado (cambios histopatológicos, inducción enzimática); en dichos estudios los NOEL estaban comprendidos entre 0,05 y 0,07 mg de HCB/kg de peso corporal al día. Las concentraciones de neurotransmisores en el hipotálamo se vieron alteradas en visones hembra sometidos a través de los alimentos a una exposición crónica de 0,16 mg de HCB/kg de peso corporal al día, y en su descendencia expuesta a lo largo de la gestación y la lactancia. En estudios subcrónicos realizados en ratas la homeostasis del calcio y la morfometría ósea se vieron afectadas con 0,7 mg de HCB/kg de peso corporal al día, pero no con 0,07 mg/kg de peso corporal al día.

La carcinogenicidad del HCB ha sido evaluada mediante varios bioensayos realizados con roedores. En hámsters mantenidos con alimentos con los que ingerían unas dosis medias de 4, 8 ó 16 mg/kg de peso corporal al día durante toda la vida, se produjeron aumentos en la incidencia de tumores de las células del hígado (hepatomas) en los dos sexos y a todas las dosis, hemangioendoteliomas hepáticos a dosis de 8-16 mg/kg de peso corporal al día, y adenomas tiroideos de los machos a la dosis mayor. La exposición alimentaria de ratones a dosis de 6, 12 y 24 mg/kg de peso corporal al día durante 120 semanas dio lugar a un aumento de la incidencia de tumores de las células del hígado (hepatomas) en ambos sexos a las dos dosis mayores (no significativo, excepto para las hembras a la dosis mayor). En ratas, la exposición *in útero*, durante la lactancia y por vía oral al HCB a través de alimentos que proporcionaban a lo largo de su vida dosis medias comprendidas entre 0,01 y 1,5 mg/kg de peso corporal al día (machos) o 1,9 mg/kg de peso corporal al día (hembras) por espacio de hasta 130 semanas *post útero* produjo a la mayor de las dosis un aumento de la incidencia de nódulos hepáticos neoplásicos y de feocromocitomas suprarrenales en las hembras y de adenomas paratiroideos en los machos. En otro estudio crónico realizado en la rata, la exposición por un periodo de hasta dos años a alimentos que proporcionaban dosis medias de HCB de 4-5 y de 8-9 mg/kg de peso corporal al día indujo aumentos de la incidencia de hepatomas y de adenomas de las células renales a ambas dosis en los dos sexos, y de carcinomas hepatocelulares, adenomas y carcinomas de las vías biliares, y feocromocitomas suprarrenales y adenomas de la corteza suprarrenal en las hembras. Se ha informado también de incidencias elevadas de tumores hepáticos en algunos estudios más limitados en los que se administraron concentraciones alimentarias únicas a grupos reducidos de ratas hembra. Además, se ha informado de que, después de una exposición alimentaria subcrónica al HCB, ratones, hámsters y ratas desarrollaron tumores en el hígado, las vías biliares, el riñón, el timo, el bazo y los ganglios linfáticos. La exposición alimentaria al HCB favoreció la inducción de tumores hepáticos por el terfenilo policlorado en el ratón y por la dietilnitrosamina en la rata.

Con excepción de los tumores renales en la rata macho (aparentemente debidos, al menos en parte, a una nefropatía por acumulación de gotas hialinas) y de los hepatomas en la rata (posible resultado de la respuesta hiperplásica a una necrosis hepatocelular), no se conocen estudios mecanísticos que hayan determinado el significado del tipo de tumores inducidos por el HCB en el caso del hombre.

El HCB tiene una escasa capacidad de inducción directa de mutaciones de los genes, lesiones cromosómicas y reparaciones del ADN. Mostró una leve actividad mutágena en un reducido número de los estudios realizados en bacterias y levaduras, aunque hay que señalar que todos esos estudios presentan limitaciones. Existen también algunos indicios de un cierto grado de unión al ADN *in vitro* e *in vivo*, aunque a niveles muy inferiores a los habituales en los carcinógenos genotóxicos.

En estudios sobre la reproducción, la exposición oral de monos a tan sólo 0,1 mg de HCB/kg de peso corporal al día durante 90 días afectó a la estructura revelada por microscopia óptica y a la ultraestructura del epitelio germinal superficial, una diana poco usual para las toxinas que afectan al ovario. Dicha dosis causó también daños ultraestructurales en las células germinales primordiales. Estos cambios específicos en tejidos-diana, para los que dosis mayores son aún más lesivas, se asocian por lo demás a un desarrollo normal del folículo, el ovocito y el embrión, lo que indica que el HCB tiene una acción específica en el ovario. La reproducción masculina sólo se vio afectada a dosis mucho mayores (entre 30 y 221 mg/kg de peso corporal al día) en estudios realizados en varias especies distintas de los primates.

La exposición de ratas y gatos, a través de la placenta o durante la lactancia, a dosis maternas comprendidas entre 3 y 4 mg/kg de peso corporal al día tuvo efectos hepatotóxicos o afectó a la supervivencia o el crecimiento de la descendencia en período de lactancia. En algunos casos, dosis iguales o superiores a ésas redujeron el tamaño de las camadas o aumentaron el número de abortos. (Los efectos nocivos en los cachorros sin destetar han sido observados más frecuentemente, y a dosis menores, que los efectos embriotóxicos o fetotóxicos.) La descendencia de visones expuestos crónicamente a sólo 1 mg de HCB/kg de alimento (aproximadamente 0,16 mg/kg de peso corporal al día) tuvo un peso reducido al nacer y presentó una mayor mortalidad hasta el destete. A pesar de que se han observado trastornos esqueléticos y renales de los fetos en algunos estudios realizados en ratas y ratones expuestos al HCB durante la gestación, dichas alteraciones o bien no estaban claramente relacionadas con el tratamiento o bien ocurrieron a dosis que eran también tóxicas para las madres. En dos estudios, uno de los cuales incluía exposición posnatal y durante la lactancia, el desarrollo neurocomportamental de las crías de rata se vio afectado por la exposición *in útero* a dosis maternas orales de 0,64 a 2,5 mg de HCB/kg de peso corporal al día.

Los resultados de varios estudios indican que el HCB afecta al sistema inmunitario. Ratas y monos expuestos a dosis entre 3 y 120 mg de HCB/kg de peso corporal al día sufrieron alteraciones histopatológicas en el timo, en el bazo y en los ganglios linfáticos o los tejidos linfoides del pulmón. La exposición crónica de perros sabuesos a 0,12 mg/kg de peso corporal al día produjo una hiperplasia nodular del tejido linfoide gástrico. En varios estudios realizados en la rata, la inmunidad humoral y, en menor grado, la celular se vieron potenciadas tras varias semanas de exposición alimentaria al HCB, mientras que la función de los macrófagos no se alteró. Una cantidad tan pequeña como 4 mg de HCB/kg de alimento (aproximadamente 0,2 mg/kg de peso corporal al día) durante la gestación, a lo largo de la lactancia y hasta las 5 semanas de edad incrementó las respuestas inmunitarias humoral y celular y provocó la acumulación de macrófagos en el tejido pulmonar de crías de rata. Por el contrario, se ha observado un efecto inmunodepresor del HCB en la mayor parte de los estudios llevados a cabo con ratones; dosis de sólo 0,5-0,6 mg/kg de peso corporal al día durante varias semanas redujeron la resistencia a la infección por *Leishmania* o a una provocación con células tumorales, disminuyeron la actividad citotóxica de los macrófagos del bazo, y redujeron la respuesta de hipersensibilidad de tipo retardado en la descendencia expuesta *in útero* y durante la lactancia. En varios estudios realizados con diversas cepas de ratas, la exposición de breve duración o subcrónica al HCB afectó a la función tiroidea, a juzgar por los reducidos niveles séricos de tiroxina total y tiroxina libre (T_4) y a menudo, en menor grado, de triyodotironina (T_3).

Efectos en el ser humano

La mayor parte de los datos acerca de los efectos del HCB en el ser humano provienen de intoxicaciones accidentales que tuvieron lugar en Turquía en los años 1955-1959, entre las que se identificaron más de 600 casos de porfiria cutánea tardía (PCT). En esa ocasión se observaron alteraciones en el metabolismo de la porfirina, lesiones dermatológicas, hiperpigmentación, hipertricosis, aumento del tamaño del hígado, de la glándula tiroides y de los ganglios linfáticos; se observaron también (aproximadamente en la mitad de los casos) osteoporosis o artritis, sobre todo en los niños. Los niños amamantados por madres expuestas al HCB como consecuencia de ese accidente desarrollaron un trastorno conocido como pembe yara (ulceración rosada), y la mayor parte murieron antes de un año. Existen también algunos indicios de que la PCT afecta a personas sometidas a una exposición relativamente alta al HCB en el lugar de trabajo o en el medio ambiente general.

Los pocos estudios epidemiológicos disponibles acerca de la incidencia de cáncer tienen un valor limitado, ya sea por lo reducido de la muestra, por la deficiente caracterización de la exposición al CHB o por la exposición a otros muchos agentes, y son insuficientes para evaluar la carcinogenicidad del HCB para el ser humano.

8. Efectos en otros organismos en el laboratorio y sobre el terreno

En los estudios realizados sobre la toxicidad aguda del HCB para los organismos acuáticos, la exposición a concentraciones comprendidas entre 1 y 17 µg/litro redujo la producción de clorofila en algas y la reproducción de protozoos ciliados, y causó mortalidad en el camarón rosado y en las quisquillas, pero no aumentó la mortalidad de peces de agua dulce o de mar. En estudios a largo plazo, el crecimiento de algas y protozoos vulnerables de agua dulce se vio afectado por una concentración de 1 µg/litro, mientras que concentraciones de aproximadamente 3 µg/litro provocaron mortalidad en anfípodos y necrosis hepática en la perca americana.

9. Evaluación de los riesgos para la salud humana y de los efectos en el medio ambiente

9.1 Efectos en la salud

El Grupo Especial llegó a la conclusión de que los datos disponibles son suficientes para establecer valores indicativos respecto a los efectos neoplásicos y no neoplásicos del HCB.

En cuanto a los efectos no neoplásicos, considerando el NOEL más bajo notificado (0,05 mg de HCB/kg de peso corporal al día), referido sobre todo a los efectos hepáticos observados a dosis mayores en estudios realizados en cerdos y ratas expuestos por vía oral, e incorporando un factor de incertidumbre de 300 (x 10 en concepto de variación interespecíes, x 10 en concepto de variación intraespecie, y x 3 en concepto de gravedad del efecto), se ha calculado una IDT de 0,17 µg/kg de peso corporal al día.

El criterio seguido en cuanto a los efectos neoplásicos se basa en la dosis tumorigénica TD_5, es decir, la ingesta asociada a un exceso del 5% en la incidencia de tumores detectada en los experimentos con animales. Considerando los resultados del bioensayo de carcinogenicidad en dos generaciones de ratas, y empleando el modelo polietápico, la TD_5 es de 0,81 mg/kg de peso corporal al día para los nódulos neoplásicos del hígado en las hembras. Habida cuenta de la insuficiencia de los datos mecanísticos, se utilizó un factor de incertidumbre de 5000 para establecer un valor indicativo, basado en criterios de salud, de 0,16 µg/kg de peso corporal al día.

9.2 Efectos en el medio ambiente

El Grupo Especial señaló que existen muy pocos estudios experimentales con los que llevar a cabo una evaluación de los riesgos para el medio ambiente. Los niveles de HCB en las aguas superficiales, excepto en unos pocos lugares extremadamente contaminados, son en general varios órdenes de magnitud inferiores a los que se supone que entrañan riesgos para los organismos acuáticos. No obstante, las concentraciones de HCB en los huevos de las aves marinas y las rapaces de algunos lugares en distintas zonas del mundo se aproximan a niveles que en la gaviota argéntea se asocian a una disminución del peso del embrión (1500 µg/kg), lo que parece indicar que el HCB puede dañar los embriones de especies de aves vulnerables. Del mismo modo, los niveles de HCB observados en peces de diversos lugares del mundo se encuentran a un orden de magnitud del nivel alimentario de 1000 µg/kg, asociado a una reducción del peso al nacer y a un aumento de la mortalidad de la descendencia en los visones. Esto parece indicar que el HCB puede tener efectos nocivos en los visones y, tal vez, en otros mamíferos que se alimentan de peces.

10. Conclusiones

a) El HCB es un producto químico persistente que se bioacumula debido a su liposolubilidad y a su resistencia a la degradación.

b) Los estudios realizados con animales han demostrado que el HCB produce cáncer y afecta a una amplia gama de sistemas de órganos, con inclusión del hígado, los pulmones, los riñones, la tiroides, los tejidos reproductivos y los sistemas nervioso e inmunitario.

c) En seres humanos sometidos a una alta exposición accidental se ha observado toxicidad sintomática, en particular porfiria cutánea tardía en niños y en adultos y mortalidad en lactantes.

d) Es necesario adoptar diversas medidas para reducir la carga ambiental de HCB.

e) Se han propuesto los siguientes valores indicativos basados en criterios de salud para la ingesta diaria total (IDT) de HCB por el ser humano: efectos no cancerígenos, 0,17 µg/kg de peso corporal/día; efectos neoplásicos, 0,16 µ/kg de peso corporal/día.

---

[a] Out of print